" *What man requires most in life*
Is for someone to make him do
What he is capable of doing. "

R. E.

Pharmacology for the
Health Professional

DANIEL E. BECKER, D.D.S.

Pharmacology for the Health Professional

RESTON PUBLISHING COMPANY, INC.
A PRENTICE-HALL COMPANY
RESTON, VIRGINIA

Library of Congress Cataloging in Publication Data

Becker, Daniel E.
  Pharmacology for the health professional.

  Includes bibliographies.
  1. Pharmacology. I. Title. [DNLM: 1. Pharmacology.
  QV 38 B395p]
  RM300.B39 1985   615'.1   84-27674
  ISBN 0-8359-5531-1

1   3   5   7   9   10   8   6   4   2

PRINTED IN THE UNITED STATES OF AMERICA

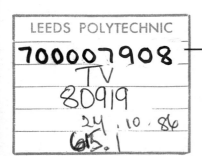

Contents

x

Contents

List of Tables

Preface

Pharmacology for the Health Professional is not intended as a text in the classical sense. Instead, it represents a philosophy of teaching fundamental principles appropriate for the undergraduate student. The goal is not to create an authoritative reference, but to teach a pharmacology course with a practical textbook.

Every health profession recognizes several texts, each dedicated to the uniqueness of that particular field of practice. Unfortunately, drugs are not so selective in their behavior. Epinephrine may be used differently by each profession but its actions and effects are common whether administered by a paramedic, nurse, respiratory therapist, or other health professional. For this reason, the basic principles of pharmacology must be common knowledge for all allied health students, regardless of their specific professional track. By necessity or curiosity, some students will require a more in-depth presentation than others and, for this reason, *Pharmacology for the Health Professional* presents both general and special information. The latter is quoted in those paragraphs marked by a vertical bar. They may be skipped over by those students who are less involved in the handling and administration of drug preparations.

Only the most fundamental principles of a drug class are presented in each chapter. The instructor may than direct the students into areas of more specific concern. Although instructors may prefer personally to select articles, source references and suggested reading lists are provided for this purpose. Some of these professional articles address pharmacological agents not discussed in the text. This is intentional. Students must be aware that they can gather current information and actually "understand the stuff" by applying their knowledge of fundamental principles and drug prototypes. For example, diltiazem is not thoroughly addressed in this text, but principles of calcium channel blockade are. That knowledge must be used to stay abreast of information on any newer members of this drug class as they become available for clinical use. The instructor may assign articles to small groups or the entire class and require that they be presented orally or handed in as written synopses. In this manner, a pharmacology course not only teaches principles of drug use, but also offers experience in library use, reading, composition, and speech.

In summary, *Pharmacology for the Health Professional* is designed as a foundation on which pharmacology instruction may be expanded into any area deemed important by the individual instructor. Each instructor is unique, and the only perfect text would be one written by that instructor. It is hoped that this particular text, combined with optional journal article review, will provide the pedagogical framework for a multitude of individualized approaches to training our health professionals.

D.E.B.

ACKNOWLEDGMENTS : It was during that first meeting of Dr Rush Elliott's comparative vertebrate anatomy class at Ohio University that my career in education was chosen. He and his able colleague, Mrs Allen, were so organized, challenging, and demanding that a total respect was unavoidable. While family pressures guided me through a rather unorthodox educational track towards the teaching profession, it was their influence that sustained my drive. And finally, I will be forever grateful to Mr Lynn Timmons, Mrs Judy Brozka and Dr Louise Katz for granting me that first opportunity to realize my goals at Sinclair College.

Pharmacology for the
Health Professional

1

Introduction and General Principles

Drugs are those chemicals which interact with living tissues to produce therapeutic and/or toxic effects. On this basis it is quite apparent that principles of pharmacology rely heavily on principles of other biological and physical sciences. Even an introductory study requires that the student have a background in anatomy, physiology, and chemistry.

There are two fundamental concepts one must grasp when commencing a course in pharmacology. First, drugs can alter only those functions that are within the capabilities of a particular tissue or cell type. (We have yet to synthesize a drug that can stimulate salivary glands to produce insulin!) Second, drugs must possess some degree of specificity in action. Otherwise, they would produce a spectrum of undesired effects overshadowing their usefulness.

NOMENCLATURE AND CLASSIFICATION

Early in its development, a drug may be referred to by a *chemical* name (N-acetyl-p-aminophenol) or by a more succinct *generic* name (acetaminophen). When the company involved is granted permission to market the drug, it assigns a *brand* name (for example, Tylenol) to the drug. The company which develops the drug is granted a patent, that is, exclusive marketing rights, for 17 years. After this time, other companies may market the generic drug using its generic name or assigning it another brand name (Acetaminophen, Datril, Tempra).

There are several methods by which drugs may be classified. Unfortunately this variety of methods may confuse the beginning student since a single drug may be described as belonging to several classes. Drugs are most typically classified according to their chemical group, their mechanism or site of action, and their primary effect(s). On this basis, the familiar drug, diazepam (Valium), may

3

be referred to as a benzodiazepine, a central nervous system (CNS) depressant, or an anxiolytic.

PHARMACOKINETICS

Pharmacokinetics deals with the absorption, distribution, metabolism, and elimination of drug molecules. It represents a very complex subject relying heavily on principles of mathematics, chemistry, and physics. A general discussion of these concepts is necessary to understand factors which determine the magnitude and the duration of drug action.

Routes of administration may be conveniently divided into two major categories, enteral and parenteral. Enteral routes include all methods in which a medication enters the gastrointestinal (GI) tract and passes through these membranes to gain entry to the circulation (absorption). By strict definition, parenteral routes would include all other methods of administration. Unfortunately, many use the word to imply "by injection." Table 1.1 offers an acceptable system of classification, although many authors vary their definitions.

Absorption is the process by which drugs enter the circulatory system. With the exception of intravascular injections, all routes require that the drug pass through layers of tissue to enter the circulation. Fundamental to this process of absorption is the drug's ability to pass through cell membranes. Since the greatest portion of any cell membrane is lipid, it follows that lipid-soluble drugs are more readily absorbed than those which are water-soluble. The absorptive process generally obeys the principles of passive diffusion.

Very small, water-soluble molecules are able to pass through tiny pores within the cell membrane. Water-soluble molecules having a molecular weight in excess of 200 cannot pass through these pores and are therefore poorly absorbed by routes other than intravascular or intramuscular injection. Ionization of the drug molecule is a major determinant of lipid solubility. Nonionized forms tend to be lipid-soluble and are more likely to be absorbed than ionized species, which are water-soluble. When drugs are described as being "polar-compounds," you may assume that they are poorly absorbed and are more efficiently administered by parenteral routes. Additionally, they are less likely to penetrate the "blood-brain" barrier and produce CNS effects.

Once the drug has been absorbed, it is distributed throughout the body by the circulatory system. At this point, the concept of *bioavailability* becomes extremely important. It refers to the amount of drug available in its active form to produce its intended effect on the target tissue. Obviously, any portion not ab-

TABLE 1.1   Routes of drug administration

Enteral	Parenteral	Topical
1. any form swallowed	1. intravenous (IV)	1. sublingual*
	2. subcutaneous (SubQ)	2. rectal*
	3. intramuscular (IM)	3. vaginal
	4. intrathecal (spinal)	4. nasal
		5. conjunctival
		6. inhalational**

*Strictly speaking, these would actually be enteral routes since oral and rectal mucosa are considered gastrointestinal components and absorption is generally intended.
**When used for general anesthesia, a systemic, rather than a local effect, is desired.

sorbed will be unavailable, but additional factors play critical roles in determining bioavailability following absorption.

Drug molecules may become stored in adipose tissue or bound to plasma protein, for example, albumin. In either case, the stored molecules are not bioavailable until they are released from storage, an event that may be delayed for hours or days following administration. An example of fat storage occurs during thiopental anesthesia. During the postoperative period, the drug is released slowly from storage sites rendering the patient sluggish and sedated, an event commonly referred to as "barbiturate hangover."

Rapid drug metabolism (biotransformation) may limit the bioavailability of an administered drug. This is especially true when one swallows an oral preparation. Following absorption, the drug must travel within the hepatic portal vein to the liver where "first-pass" metabolism may destroy a significant quantity of the drug before any reaches the general circulation and the target tissues.

Most biotransformation reactions occur in the liver. Here the hepatocytes synthesize many enzyme systems (microsomal enzymes) and conjugates, which may render drug molecules inactive and/or water-soluble, facilitating their renal excretion.

One must not conclude that all biotransformations occur within the liver since they may actually occur anywhere in the body. Neither should one conclude that the products of these reactions (metabolites) are always harmless and inactive and ready for excretion. In some cases, the metabolites are therapeutically useful while in other cases they may be toxic. For example, the hepatotoxicity attributed to acetaminophen (Tylenol and so forth) overdose is actually due to one of its metabolites, not the parent compound.[1]

The relationship of the vascular supply to the brain and the fetus represents a barrier to the distribution of drugs to these tissues. The so-called "blood-brain" and "placental" barriers limit the diffusion of water-soluble drugs and thus allow greater bioavailability of lipid-soluble drugs within the central nervous system and the fetus.

> The blood-brain barrier is actually caused by the tight junctions between endothelial cells comprising the capillaries within the brain. The presence of various glial cells and myelin also impedes diffusion of water-soluble molecules. Within the placenta, the fetal blood is separated from the maternal circulation not only by the endothelium but by a layer of columnar-shaped cells termed the "trophoblastic" layer (Figure 1.1A and 1.1B).

Figure 1.1A   Blood-Brain Barrier
In order to affect the neurons within the central nervous system, a drug molecule must diffuse through the capillary endothelium, glial layers, and, in some cases, myelin coating the axonal fiber. The capillary endothelium is especially significant since the individual cells are tightly joined together (compared to other capillary systems where the cells are very loosely joined). Therefore, drug molecules must pass through the cell membranes, not between the endothelial cells. The total of these factors is abstractly referred to as the "blood-brain barrier."

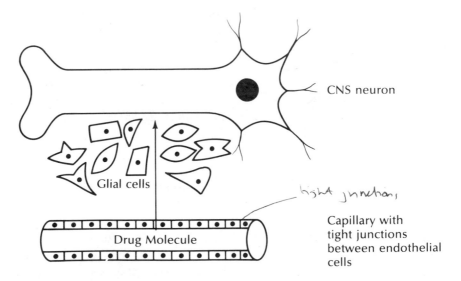

Figure 1.1B   Placental Barrier

Maternal blood empties into sinuses (S) which surround capillary villi formed by the fetal vessels. Drug molecules must diffuse through a layer of cuboidal cells (Trophoblasts) if they are to enter the fetal circulation. These trophoblastic cells are the major component of what is referred to as the "placental barrier."

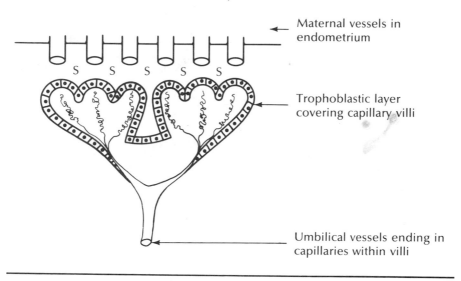

Maternal vessels in endometrium

Trophoblastic layer covering capillary villi

Umbilical vessels ending in capillaries within villi

From a quantitative standpoint, the kidney is the major route of elimination for parent compounds and their metabolites. In contrast to absorption, water solubility enhances the excretion by this route. Should biotransformation reactions fail to alter lipid solubility, reabsorption through the renal tubules will provide for redistribution throughout the body. Eventually, however, water-soluble metabolites will be formed, which are eliminated in urine. Although renal excretion is the major route of drug excretion, one must bear in mind that any human excrement may serve as a vehicle for elimination. Mammary excretion, although small by quantitative standards, is hardly insignificant to the nursing infant.

Figure 1.2 (see overleaf) illustrates the major features of pharmacokinetic principles. The student may consult a more detailed text for further information regarding these concepts.

PHARMACODYNAMICS

The physiological and biochemical effects actually produced on living tissues is considered under the title of pharmacodynamics. Thus far we have followed a

Figure 1.2
Hypothetical pharmacokinetic pattern following PO, IV, or IM administration. Notice reduced amount required when administering drug by the parenteral route as compared to PO.

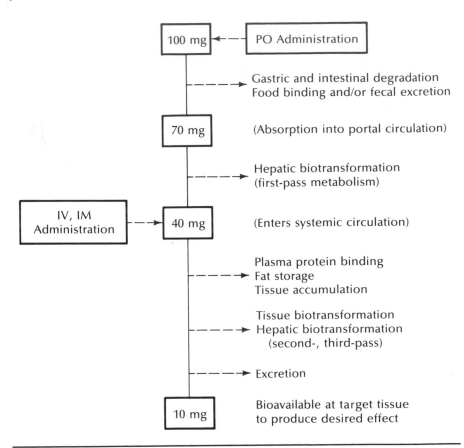

drug from administration to excretion without examining its actual effect on the intended target organs. A complete analysis of these mechanisms would be inappropriate, but the fundamental fact is that drugs can only facilitate or inhibit the normal functions of a particular tissue.

⟶   The most common mechanism by which drugs exert their effects on living tissues is by interaction with specific macromolecular components of cells. These specific molecules are called *receptors* and may be found in great numbers on cell membranes or on any cytoplasmic organelle. Drugs that bind to a specific receptor are claimed to have *receptor affinity* and may or may not generate a biochemical response by the cell, that is, possess *intrinsic activity*. Drugs possessing receptor affinity and intrinsic activity are called *agonists*, while those having affinity for the receptor but unable to produce intrinsic activity are called *antagonists* (see Figure 1.3). While the latter do not produce an actual effect on the cell, they are useful clinically for their ability to prevent the action produced by the agonist for the receptor.

> The human body did not evolve receptors to interact with drug molecules. Rather they serve to interact exquisitely with endogenous chemicals for the orchestration of normal physiological processes. By interacting with these receptors, such exogenous chemicals as drugs are able to alter normal body functions. For example, in 1973 the opiate receptors with which narcotic analgesics interact to produce their many effects were identified. What excited pharmacologists most, however, was the challenge to identify the endogenous substance (ligand) for which the receptors were designed. Certainly we were not born with receptors for morphine! In 1975 the endorphin ligands were identified and will be addressed further in Chapter 11.

Figure 1.3   Receptor Mechanism of Drug Action

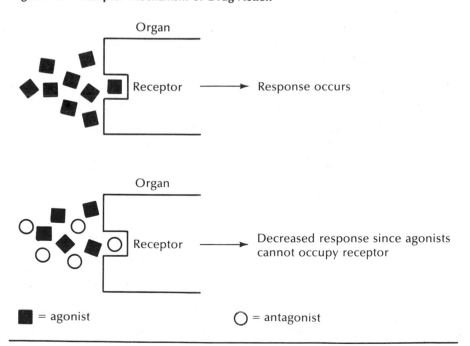

Acetylcholine is an endogenous agonist released by many neurons. When released by those neurons supplying salivary glands, it attaches to specific receptors on the cell membranes of glandular cells called muscarinic receptors. This interaction between acetylcholine and the muscarinic receptor results in salivation. The drug, atropine, is a muscarinic receptor antagonist which denies acetylcholine access to the receptor. The result is salivary inhibition (see Figure 1.4).

(A)

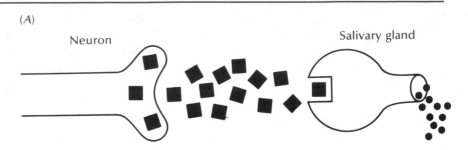

Figure 1.4
A. Normally, salivary excretion is stimulated by acetylcholine (■).
B. This process is inhibited following the administration of the receptor antagonist, atropine (O).

(B)

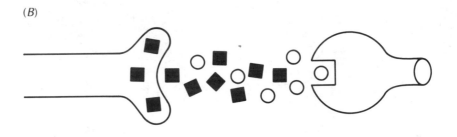

A similar mechanism by which drugs produce their effects is *enzyme interference*. All body processes require chemical reactions catalyzed by enzymes. Drugs may compete for these enzymes as false substrates, thus rendering a critical chemical pathway deficient in its regulatory enzyme. It is possible to view this mechanism as a further example of the receptor concept discussed above. If we adopt this viewpoint, the enzyme is actually the receptor, the competing substrate (drug) is the receptor antagonist, and the normal endogenous substrate is the agonist (see Figure 1.5).

(A)

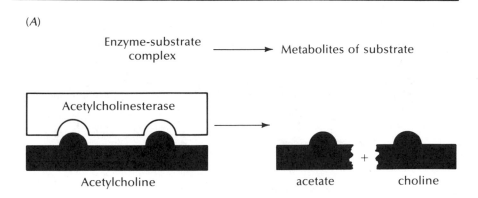

Figure 1.5
In A above, the substrate (acetylcholine) may be viewed as an agonist reacting with its receptor (the enzyme acetylcholinesterase). The result is the formation of acetate and choline. In B below, the false substrate (neostigmine) may then be viewed as an antagonist that fits the receptor, but since the agonist (acetylcholine) cannot occupy the receptor, no reaction occurs.

(B)

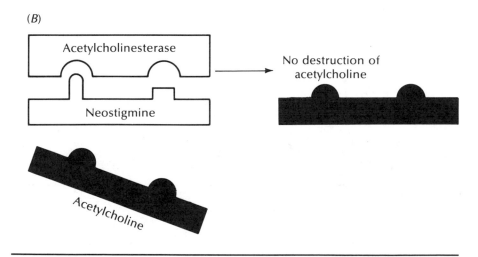

Although several nonreceptor mechanisms could be discussed, let us conclude with the concept of "counterfeit incorporation." In this mechanism, the molecular structure of a particular drug closely resembles that of a molecule within a critical metabolic sequence. Incorporation of the "counterfeit" (drug) into the pathway interrupts the sequence and results in an inferior final product.

This mechanism is utilized by many chemotherapeutic agents, including the sulfonamide antimicrobial agents (see Figure 1.6).

Figure 1.6
Sulfonamides resemble paraminobenzoic acid (PABA) in structure. Certain bacteria erroneously utilize the sulfonamide to synthesize their DNA. Thus the sulfonamide "counterfeits" itself into this metabolic pathway.

Normal Sequence

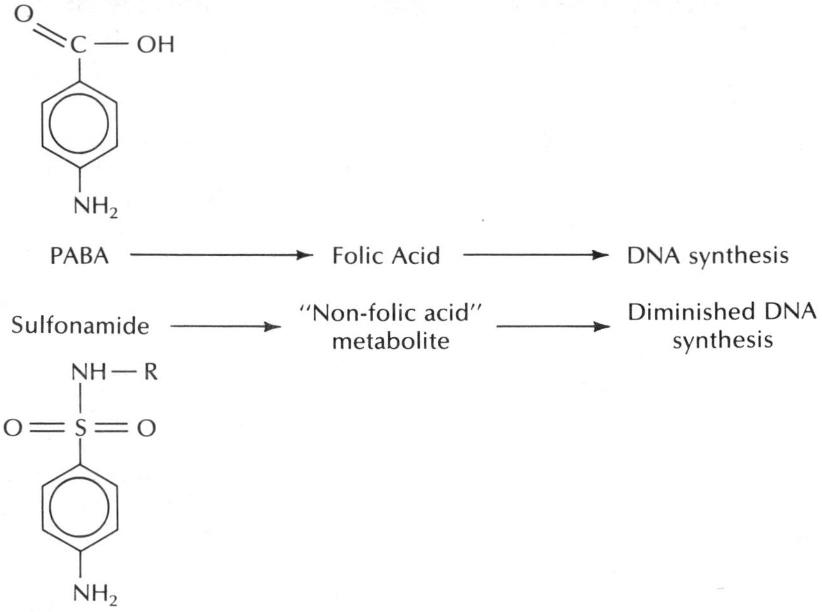

PABA $\longrightarrow$ Folic Acid $\longrightarrow$ DNA synthesis

Sulfonamide $\longrightarrow$ "Non-folic acid" metabolite $\longrightarrow$ Diminished DNA synthesis

---

ACTIONS, EFFECTS, AND INDICATIONS

Before we continue further with our study, certain definitions must be established. The *action* of a drug describes the mechanism by which it affects the tissues. It then follows that drug *effects* are those physiological changes resulting from a drug's action. Drug *indications* are the patient conditions for which the drug is administered. If we use propranolol (Inderal) as an example, the correct use of these terms will be evident:

Indication: Tachycardia, hypertension, others.
Effect: Decreased heart rate and force of contraction.
Action: Acts as a receptor antagonist at cardiac beta receptors.

It is typical for a drug to produce several physiological changes or effects, and therefore we must categorize them as primary or secondary. The effect that is desired must be considered the *primary effect*. Any additional effects are *secondary* and may be further categorized as minor or major. Many terms are used by clinicians when describing secondary effects, such as side, untoward, toxic, and adverse. Since an exact method of classification is arbitrary, the following seems logical: secondary effects that may threaten life are considered "adverse" or "toxic," while those that are merely bothersome are referred to as "side effects." It is not uncommon to interchange primary and secondary effects, depending on the effect desired. The effects produced by atropine are numerous, including salivary inhibition, increased heart rate, and decreased GI motility. If we administered atropine preoperatively to reduce secretions, the remaining effects may be considered secondary. However, if administered to a bradycardic patient, increased heart rate must be considered the primary effect while reduced secretions must now be included with the secondary effects. The essence of this concept is that secondary effects must not always be considered undesirable.

POSOLOGY AND DOSE-RESPONSE

The study of dosage (posology) is potentially a very complex subject based on pharmacokinetic and pharmacodynamic principles. Since this is an introductory text, only those concepts relevant to clinical practice will be discussed.

Efficacy is the term used to describe the maximum effect a drug may produce. *Potency* refers to the amount of drug required to produce efficacy. This may be illustrated by the dose-response curve seen in Figure 1.7A. From this graph, one can see that ibuprofen has greater potency and efficacy in relieving pain than acetaminophen. From Figure 1.7B you can deduce that nalbuphine and morphine have equal potency in relieving moderately severe pain, but morphine has greater analgesic efficacy since it may relieve severe pain at doses greater than 10 mg, whereas nalbuphine will not achieve this effect even by doubling its dose. Of these two concepts, potency and efficacy, the latter is most significant in selecting a drug for a patient. The amount is not the critical factor—the maximum effect is! Figure 1.7 overleaf illustrates both factors.

During the development of a drug, dosage is first established in laboratory animals. The dose that produces the desired response in 50 percent of the animals is designated as the ED_{50} (median effective dose) and that which proves lethal for 50 percent of the animals is the LD_{50} (lethal dose). In attempting to extrapolate these doses to humans, difficulty arises from the limited number of patients willing to participate—especially for the LD_{50} portion of the study! For this reason, TD (toxic dose) is substituted for LD; and pharmacologists attempt to establish the effective dose for the greatest number of patients possible, for example, ED_{99},

14

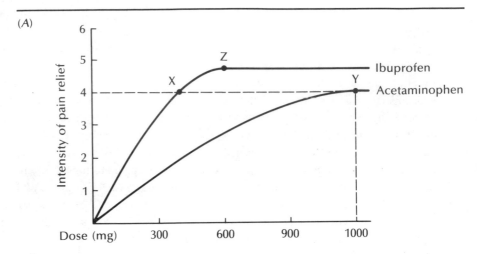

Figure 1.7
A. In graph A, 600 mg provides ibuprofen's maximum capability in relieving pain (efficacy). Increasing its dose to 900 mg offers no improvement in the intensity of pain relieved. To provide pain relief at level 4, ibuprofen requires a dose of 400 mg (X). To achieve this same level of relief, acetaminophen requires a dose of 1000 mg (Y). Therefore, we conclude that ibuprofen possesses greater potency than acetaminophen. Since ibuprofen is also capable of producing a greater intensity of pain relief (Z), it also possesses greater efficacy.
B. In graph B, morphine and nalbuphine are equal in potency for relieving pain of intensity values through 8 .(x) However, increasing the dose past 10 mg illustrates morphine's superior efficacy (Z). Furthermore, if you compare the drugs in graph B to those in graph A you may conclude that morphine and nalbuphine are more potent and efficacious than either ibuprofen or acetaminophen.

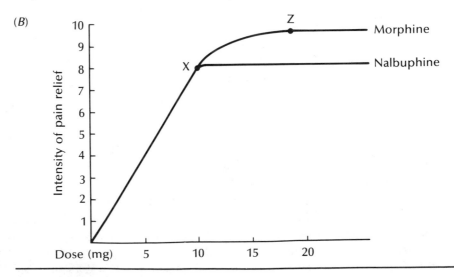

and the dose at which the fewest number of patients experience significant toxic effects, for example, TD_1. A margin of safety called the *therapeutic index* can then be calculated by dividing the LD_{50} by the ED_{50} in animals and the TD_1 by the ED_{99} in humans. The greater the therapeutic index, the greater the margin of safety. If we look at the drug in Figure 1.8, we find its therapeutic index to be 20. Theoretically, the effective dose could be increased 19 times without reaching the lethal dose. (However, we are not so naive as to recommend this practice.) The practical application of the therapeutic index may be seen by considering its value as "2" for the digitalis glycosides. Merely doubling the recommended dose is likely to result in serious toxicity to our patient.

Figure 1.8
In the above dose-response curves we see that 99 percent of the patients receive a beneficial effect with a dose of 5 mg. However 1 percent of the patients experience significant toxic effects with a dose of 100 mg. By dividing the TD1 (100 mg) by the ED99 (5 mg) we find the therapeutic index to be 20.

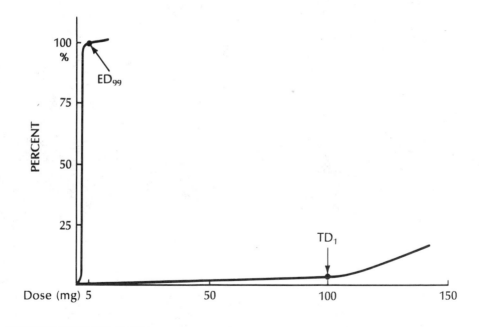

Many factors are considered when selecting a dosage for a given patient. Most drugs have a therapeutic index greater than 10, and dosages recommended in the *Physician's Desk Reference* (PDR) are generally acceptable. If more precise dosage is desired, it is generally calculated in relation to the patient's weight, for example, milligrams per kilogram of body weight. In more critical situations the dosage may be titrated intravenously with frequent blood samples taken to establish a specific blood level, for example, mcg per milliliter of blood.

Figure 1.9
In this prescription, twenty 600 mg tablets of ibuprofen are being ordered, and the patient is to take one tablet every four hours as needed.

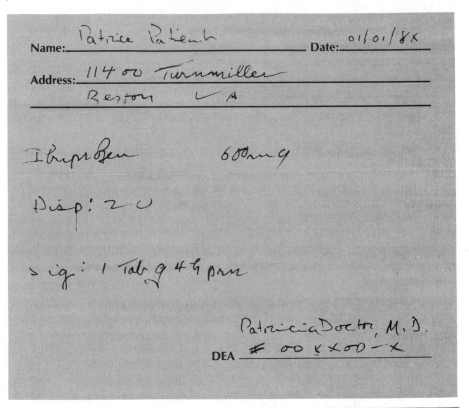

Medication orders are generally written in a patient's chart or on a prescription form and typically follow the format in Figure 1.9. Keep in mind that the format in this example does not obey all the principles of prescription writing recommended by many texts. Instead, it represents the most common format you are likely to encounter during your clinical practice. Prescriptions are written by hurried clinicians, seldom by textbook authors. Table 1.2 lists the commonly employed Latin abbreviations used in prescription orders.

TABLE 1.2   Latin abbreviations commonly employed in prescription orders

Abbreviation	Term	Interpretation
p.c.	post cibum	after meals
a.c.	ante cibum	before meals
ad lib.	ad libitum	at pleasure, freely
b.i.d.	bis in die	twice a day
t.i.d.	ter in die	three times daily
q.i.d.	quater in die	four times daily
h.	hora	hour
q.	quaque	every
c̄	cum	with
s̄	sine	without
h.s.	hora somni	at bedtime
stat.	statim	immediately
p.r.n.	pro re nata	as needed

DRUG INTERACTIONS

When two or more drugs are taken concurrently by a patient, interactions between the drugs are possible. These interactions may result from a variety of mechanisms and may be useful or undesirable.

Two drugs may react chemically with one another at the molecular level. The anticoagulant effects of heparin may be reversed by administering protamine. This interaction constitutes a classical acid-base neutralization reaction and certainly represents a useful drug interaction.

More commonly, drug interactions involve the production of additive or subtractive effects on the patient. Additive effects produced by concurrent administration may be collectively referred to as drug enhancement. Terms used to describe enhancement interactions are summation, synergism, and potentiation. While each of these terms represents a distinct mechanism of interaction, we will not dwell on their distinct differences since they tend to be used synonymously by most clinicians.

> Summation or addition is said to occur when two drugs taken concurrently produce the same effect as would have occurred had you doubled the dose of either. Synergism and potentiation are used to describe an enhanced effect greater than that seen in summation.[2]

All medications capable of producing CNS depression will enhance one another if taken concurrently and will result in a greater degree of sedation than if taken individually. While this represents an undesired interaction in patients combining sedatives with alcoholic beverages, enhancement is useful when combining sedatives with narcotics as preoperative medications. Subtractive or, more commonly, antagonistic interactions are seen when taking a CNS depressant concurrently with a CNS stimulant. The actual outcome of this interaction is seldom predictable and seldom, if ever, useful.

A significant potential for interaction occurs when taking drugs which alter hepatic microsomal enzyme activity. Some drugs stimulate microsomal enzyme activity (enzyme induction) while others may actually inhibit these enzymes or other aspects of hepatic biotransformation. Patients taking such medications will then require an adjustment in dosage of any additional medications which undergo significant hepatic biotransformation. A prime example of this concept can be illustrated with phenobarbital, an established microsomal enzyme inducer. A patient taking phenobarbital to prevent grand mal seizures may require higher doses of other medications, since these drugs will be more rapidly biotransformed in this setting of increased microsomal activity. Conversely, the dose must then be reduced should the phenobarbital therapy be discontinued. This dosage problem is especially significant if the drugs considered have a low therapeutic index. Such would be the case with warfarin, an anticoagulant. In the presence of phenobarbital, higher than normal warfarin doses will be required to maintain a proper anticoagulant effect. However, if the patient discontinues the phenobarbital, microsomal enzyme activity will decrease and warfarin levels may then increase to the point that spontaneous hemorrhage may occur.

DRUG ABUSE

The issue of drug abuse is a popular topic of discussion for members of all professions. While favorite locations for these heated debates are numerous, these are best conducted in well-designed clinical laboratories such as the favorite college tavern. Other than religion, few subjects are discussed by so many with such self-proclaimed omniscience. Since most disagreement arises from a difference in use of fundamental terms,[3] let us begin with a few definitions that are accepted by some, totally unacceptable to others, but, most importantly, are as acceptable as any.

The term *addiction* has little if any physiological or pharmacological basis. It is a term germane to the study of psychology and implies "compulsive, drug-seeking behavior." In contrast, there are putative models for *drug dependence*.

Addiction—compulsive, drug-seeking behavior—may then be viewed as alterable by degree of dependence, as well as a multitude of personality and social factors.

Drug dependence is routinely categorized into psychological and physical subtypes, each having proposed pharmacological mechanisms for their development. It is claimed that both result in an uncomfortable "abstinence syndrome" when the drug is abruptly withdrawn. Their distinction lies within the nature of these withdrawal symptoms. Evidence of physical dependence exists when the symptoms of withdrawal resemble physiological effects the opposite of those produced by the drug implicated. In this regard, physical dependence to opioids differs from that seen with barbiturates. If withdrawal symptoms do not clearly fall within this characterization, the dependence is designated as being psychological. Further complicating the issue is the fact that many people still consider physical dependence necessary for addiction to occur—despite the fact that most "dried-out" patients return to their drug-seeking behavior. This "return-to-the-streets" behavior must be attributed to psychological factors and illustrates the inconsistent relationship of dependence to addiction. To avoid this semantic issue, some experts propose that we eliminate physical and psychological distinctions, as well as which drugs are capable of producing each type. By doing so, we may then classify patients as suffering from opioid dependence, barbiturate dependence, amphetamine dependence, and so on.

Tolerance is said to exist when increased doses are required to produce the same effects formerly produced by lower doses of a given drug. Various pharmacological mechanisms have been proposed for the development of tolerance. While it typically exists in addicted patients, it should not be considered as a primary cause for drug-seeking behavior.

In summary, addiction is a complex behavior pattern which may be influenced by social, psychological, and perhaps physical components. Although dependence and tolerance are produced pharmacologically and are often present with addiction, they must not be considered the major etiological factors.

REFERENCES

1. **Barker, J. D., et al.** 1977. Chronic excessive acetaminophen rise and liver damage. *Annals of Internal Medicine* 87:299.

2. **Goth, A.** 1981. *Medical Pharmacology*. 10th ed. St. Louis: C. V. Mosby, p. 50.

3. **Newman, R. G.** 1983. The need to redefine "addiction." *New England Journal of Medicine* 308:1096–1098.

2

Review of
the Peripheral Nervous System

THE NERVE IMPULSE

All cell membranes have several things in common. The most notable similarity is that all cell membranes are semipermeable; that is, they allow certain molecules or ions to pass through while restricting others. Neurons are cells and, therefore, possess this same membrane characteristic. While at rest, neuronal membranes are relatively impermeable to sodium ions and slightly permeable to potassium ions. As a result, one finds sodium concentrated extracellularly (see Figure 2.1A). An energy-dependent mechanism called the sodium-potassium pump continuously transports these ions to their respective locations (see Figure 2.1B). Since there is a higher concentration of positive ions extracellularly, a potential difference in electrical charge exists between the inside and the outside of the neuronal membrane, that is, the outside is more positive, and the inside is negative. It is this condition that is commonly referred to as the neuron's *resting membrane potential*. See Figure 2.1 (overleaf) and Figure 2.2A.

> One should not assume that anions exist only intracellularly or that cations exist only extracellularly. Actually, there are equal amounts of anions on both sides of the cell membrane (150mEq/L). The difference in charge is credited to selective membrane permeability to cations and the sodium-potassium pump. The resting membrane is impermeable to sodium, thus assuring sodium's extracellular concentration. However, the membrane is permeable to potassium, thus permitting potassium to diffuse from its intracellular concentration, adding to the positive charge on the membrane's external surface. Following membrane excitation, it is the sodium-potassium pump mechanism that establishes the extracellular concentration of sodium and the intracellular concentration of potassium.[1]

21

(A)

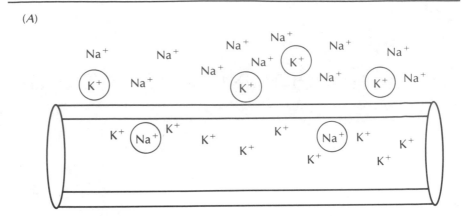

Figure 2.1   Resting Membrane Potential

A. The outside of the cell membrane is more positively charged than the inside because of the preponderance of positive ions.

B. The sodium-potassium pump ejects sodium ions from the cell. They remain in this extracellular location because the cell membrane is relatively impermeable to sodium. The pump attempts to maintain K+ intracellularly, but since the membrane is permeable to potassium, it tends to diffuse outward adding to the positive nature of the membrane's external surface.

(B)

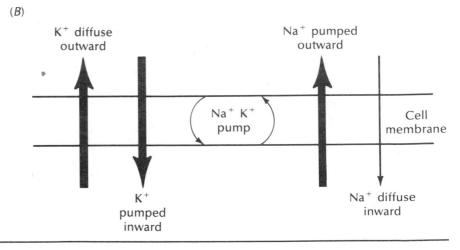

If we stimulate a neuron, its membrane becomes briefly permeable to sodium, and these positive ions diffuse into the cell causing a rapid reversal in electrical charge. This process is called *depolarization* (see Figure 2.2B).

This localized influx of sodium acts as a stimulus to the adjacent area of the membrane to become permeable to sodium, and it too begins to depolarize. This depolarization is self-propagating and continues along the entire length of the

23
The Nerve Impulse

Figure 2.2
A. Resting membrane potential.
B. Following stimulus, the cell membrane becomes permeable to Na+ ions. As they diffuse into the cell, their positive charge produces a reversal of the resting potential.
C. As soon as sodium enters the cell, the sodium-potassium pump returns sodium to the exterior and potassium to the interior. Since the membrane remains permeable to potassium, its outward diffusion finally reestablishes the resting membrane potential, that is, repolarization occurs.

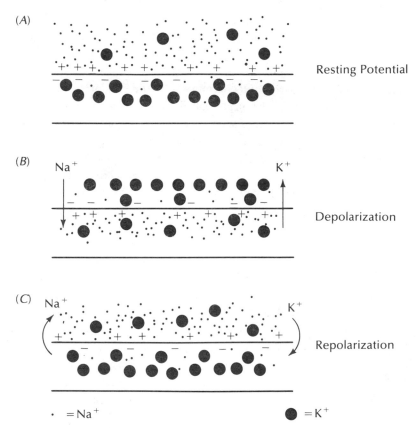

membrane. It is often referred to as the *action potential*, or *nerve impulse*. However, as soon as sodium enters the cell (depolarization), the membrane again becomes impermeable to sodium. Now the sodium-potassium pump transports sodium outwardly and potassium inwardly. Since the membrane remains somewhat permeable to potassium, these cations will diffuse outwardly until their concentration is such that the resting membrane potential is reestablished. This repolarization is illustrated in Figure 2.2C.

This nerve impulse is typical of both motor and sensory neurons and may be initiated by a wide variety of chemical, thermal, and mechanical stimuli. In motor neurons we find that the impulse is initiated by chemical stimuli within the central nervous system. These chemical stimuli represent the essence of neuropharmacology. It is important to keep in mind that although we illustrate a single nerve fiber, a nerve is actually comprised of many, many axons, all carrying these impulses.

SYNAPTIC TRANSMISSION

In a typical motor neuron, the impulse is initiated by a chemical stimulation of the neuronal cell body located within the brain or the spinal cord. The impulse travels down the length of the neuron until it reaches the end of the neuron, called the terminal. Located within the terminal are little sacs or packets called *vesicles*. These vesicles contain chemicals called *neurotransmitters*. When the impulse reaches the terminal, it stimulates the vesicles to release their neurotransmitter. The neurotransmitter then diffuses across the *synaptic cleft* (gap between the nerve ending and the muscle), attaches to a *receptor* on the muscle, and initiates a series of complex chemical events leading to muscle contraction. These receptors will take on an added significance later in this text (see Figure 2.3).

It is presently thought that the impulse reaching the neuronal terminal permits extracellular calcium ions to enter the terminal. This calcium influx in some manner initiates the release of neurotransmitter substance from the storage vesicles. (This concept is supported by the fact that low calcium levels result in a marked decrease in neurotransmitter release.) Once released, the neurotransmitter diffuses across the synaptic cleft and interacts with a specific molecule in the membrane of the muscle cell (receptor). This chemical interaction alters the muscle membrane's permeability to sodium, resulting in depolarization of the muscle cell. Following this depolarization, calcium is released from intracellular storage depots, and contraction occurs.[2]

The mechanism of action of many drugs depends on their ability to imitate or block the actions of neurotransmitters. For this reason, it is important to learn the various chemicals that function in neurotransmission. You will recall from anatomy and physiology that there are five motor endings or synaptic locations at which neurotransmitters can be released:

1. At the end of voluntary or somatic neurons, which supply skeletal muscle, the neurotransmitter is *acetylcholine* (ACh).

Figure 2.3   Synaptic Transmission

A. When the impulse reaches the nerve ending, a chemical substance called neurotransmitter (NT) is released. The NT then diffuses across the synaptic cleft and attaches to the membrane of the innervated structure producing either an excitatory or inhibitory response.

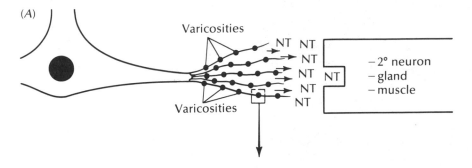

B. The neurotransmitter is stored in saclike structures called vesicles located within the varicosities of the neuronal endings. These vesicles release the NT when the neural impulse arrives at the ending.

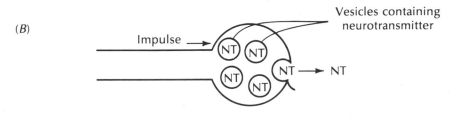

2. At the end of preganglionic parasympathetic neurons, the neurotransmitter is ACh.

3. At the end of postganglionic parasympathetic neurons, the neurotransmitter is ACh.

4. At the end of preganglionic sympathetic neurons, the neurotransmitter is ACh.

5. At the end of postganglionic sympathetic neurons, the neurotransmitter is *norepinephrine* (NE) (see Figure 2.4).

As you can see, acetylcholine is the neurotransmitter released at all motor nerve endings except postganglionic sympathetic neurons; these neurons release norepinephrine from their vesicles.

Figure 2.4 Neurotransmitters
A. Voluntary motor neurons, which innervate skeletal muscle, release acetylcholine (ACh) as their neurotransmitter.
B. Parasympathetic pathways release acetylcholine from both preganglionic and postganglionic endings.
C. Sympathetic pathways release acetylcholine from their preganglionic endings but release norepinephrine (NE) from their postganglionic endings.

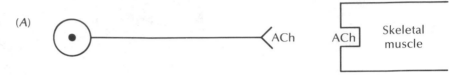

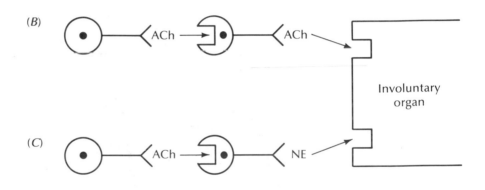

Although we say that voluntary nerves cause skeletal muscles to contract, you must now realize that *acetylcholine* causes the muscle to contract. The nerve is merely a telephone line through which the brain can control the release of *acetylcholine*. Likewise, we say that sympathetic nerves cause the heart to speed up while actually it is *norepinephrine* that causes the rate increase. The sympathetic neurons are just the telephone lines through which the brain can control the heart rate. Your next question might be, "What terminates the effect of these neurotransmitters?" Certainly they cannot last forever, or muscle activity would never stop. The effects of acetylcholine are immediately terminated by the enzyme *acetylcholinesterase* (AChE). The effect of norepinephrine is terminated in two manners. First, it may be altered by two enzymes—*monoamine oxidase* (MAO) and *catechol-o-methyltransferase* (COMT). Second, and of most importance, the nerve endings are able to "re-uptake" the released norepinephrine and salvage it for reuse. The mechanism by which this re-uptake phenomenon occurs is poorly understood, but does provide significant termination of norepinephrine, as well as of drugs similar in chemical structure. This concept will be discussed further in Chapter 4.

AUTONOMIC CONTROL

It has been stated that the function of voluntary or somatic motor neurons is to stimulate the contraction of skeletal muscles. The neurotransmitter released by these neurons, ACh, is the actual stimulus; and the release of this neurotransmitter is under our voluntary control. In contrast, the *autonomic nervous system* is comprised of neurons over which we have no conscious control. This system has two divisions; the *sympathetic* and the *parasympathetic* divisions. Each pathway is actually composed of two neurons, with each neuron releasing a neurotransmitter at its terminal ending (see Figure 2.4).

In basic anatomy and physiology it is common to perceive that the sympathetic division produces "fight-or-flight" responses while the parasympathetic division produces those responses required during periods of "conservation." This explanation unfortunately implies that sympathetic neurons stimulate while the parasympathetic neurons relax.

This concept is further nurtured by using the heart as the exemplary organ in which the sympathetics stimulate and the parasympathetics relax. Furthermore, it is often assumed that all organs receive both types of neurons, which is again a misconception. The above concepts are acceptable for understanding basic human anatomy and physiology but are totally inadequate for proper understanding of autonomic pharmacology.

Sympathetic neurons cause our heart and smooth muscles* to perform functions that will help us during periods of fight or flight. Parasympathetic neurons cause our heart and smooth muscle to perform those functions appropriate during periods of conservation. Imagine the following situation: You are walking alone, down a city street, when suddenly a grizzly bear starts chasing you. Yes, this is definitely fight or flight. With the help of the information in the chart on the next page, let us examine what must happen to various organs to help you escape this monster.

---

*Realize that smooth muscle is found in all involuntary structures except the heart; for example, blood vessels, glands, and urinary bladder.

Organs	Sympathetic Action
Heart	Rate and force increases to pump more blood.
Pupil	Dilates so you can see better.
Lungs	Bronchial muscle must relax so bronchi are dilated to allow greater volume of air exchange.
Arteries within skeletal muscles	Dilate to allow more blood to nourish skeletal muscle cells.
Other arteries	Constrict to increase pressure and channel blood to dilated skeletal arteries.
Urinary and GI sphincters	Constrict. This is no time to be going to the bathroom.
Peristalsis	Reduced. This is not the time for digesting a double cheeseburger.

The above actions are a result of sympathetic innervation to these organs. Notice that some involve stimulation while others involve relaxation. Now imagine this: You are sitting in your backyard listening to the radio and grilling hamburgers. Let us examine what happens to the same organs discussed above:

Organs	Parasympathetic Action
Heart	Rate decreases. There isn't a reason to hurry.
Pupil	Constricts. You don't need to see that well.
Lungs	Constrict the bronchioles. You don't need such a large volume of air.
Arteries	No significant control present. This is an exception to the rule of dual innervation.
Urinary and GI sphincters	Relax. You can now go to the bathroom if you want.
Peristalsis	Stimulate. So you can eat and digest the hamburgers.

All of these actions are functions of the parasympathetic division. Notice that again, some involve stimulation and some involve relaxation. There is no need to memorize the autonomic control of all the organs and structures of the body. All you have to do is name a structure and think: "What should it do during fight or flight?" Whatever the answer, sympathetic neurons cause this response and, provided there is dual control, parasympathetics produce the opposite response. In closing, test yourself with this question. What is the autonomic control of the urinary bladder? (Hint: What *should* the bladder do in a fight-or-flight situation?)

> In the above situation concerning the urinary bladder, you should have deduced that sympathetics inhibit while parasympathetics stimulate. This may seem disputable since we know that voiding often occurs during frightening situations. Although most organs receive dual autonomic innervation, seldom are the two divisions exactly equal in their influence on an organ. Generally speaking, the division that performs the stimulatory effect on the organ is the dominant innervation and, if both divisions fire simultaneously, as is the case in many fright situations, the dominant division wins. Another concept that may be puzzling you is the fact that the neurotransmitters, acetylcholine and norepinephrine, may stimulate or relax the same type of tissue—namely smooth muscle. For example, ACh stimulates smooth muscle of the GI wall but relaxes the smooth muscle of the GI sphincters. This is due to the fact that, upon interacting with a receptor on a given cell, two membrane potentials may be produced on this effector cell. An excitatory postsynaptic potential (EPSP) occurs when the receptor activation produces a depolarization of the effector cell membrane. This obviously results in the contraction of the muscle (effector). An inhibitory postsynaptic potential (IPSP) produces a hyperpolarization of the effector cell membrane. When this occurs, the effector cell membrane is stabilized and actually resists depolarization.[3]

If the content of this chapter remains somewhat confusing, you would do well to reread the entire chapter. You must master these basic concepts of normal neurophysiology before you can expect to grasp the content of the next two chapters.

REFERENCES

1. Guyton, A. C. 1980. *Textbook of Medical Physiology*. 6th ed. Philadelphia: W. B. Saunders, pp. 106–110.

2. Cooper, J. R., et al. 1978. *The Biochemical Basis of Neuropharmacology*. 3rd ed. New York: Oxford University Press, pp. 142–143.

3. Goodman, L. S., and Gilman, A. 1980. *The Pharmacological Basis of Therapeutics*. 6th ed. New York: Macmillan, pp. 66–67.

3

Cholinergic and Anticholinergic Drugs

The essence of neuropharmacology is based on simulation and antagonism of the neurotransmitters already described in Chapter 2. All nerves that release acetylcholine as a neurotransmitter are referred to as *cholinergic nerves*. You should now be able to name four cholinergic nerves (see Figure 2.4 in Chapter 2):

1. Voluntary or somatic motor
2. Preganglionic sympathetic
3. Preganglionic parasympathetic
4. Postganglionic parasympathetic

With few exceptions, postganglionic sympathetic neurons release norepinephrine and are therefore classified as "adrenergic." This concept will be further explained in Chapter 4.

CHOLINERGIC DRUGS AND RECEPTORS

A cholinergic drug is one that simulates the actions of cholinergic nerves. Stated more appropriately, a *cholinergic drug* is one that simulates the effects produced by *acetylcholine*. For example, a cholinergic drug such as methacholine will produce the following cholinergic effects:

1. Skeletal muscle contraction
2. Decrease in heart rate
3. Pupil constriction
4. Bronchial constriction
5. Salivary and GI gland secretion

Notice that these effects are identical to those produced by voluntary and parasympathetic nerves. From this information, it should be apparent that cholinergic drugs may produce a phenomenal number of body responses.

Based on their mechanism of action, cholinergic drugs may be classified as direct-acting or indirect-acting. Those classified as direct-acting exert their effects by functioning as agonists on cholinergic receptors located on structures supplied by parasympathetic nerves (smooth muscle, cardiac muscle, glands). It may be stated that they imitate the effects of parasympathetic nerves, and therefore they may be referred to as "parasympathomimetic agents." Of equal significance is the fact that most are not substrates for acetylcholinesterase, thus explaining their prolonged effect when compared to acetylcholine.

Following its release from the synaptic vesicles, the acetylcholine attaches to a receptor site on the muscle or effector resulting in an "effect." In the body we find two types of cholinergic receptors. This is to say, two types of receptors will respond to acetylcholine. Due to the specific cholinergic receptor affinity of muscarine (found in mushrooms) and nicotine, these receptors are referred to as *muscarinic* receptors and *nicotinic* receptors. Muscarinic receptors are located on all involuntary effectors—that is, effectors that receive autonomic innervation (cardiac, smooth muscle glands). When acetylcholine or muscarinic drugs occupy these receptors, the response is as if parasympathetic nerves activated them. For example, the heart slows, the pupils constrict, the bronchials constrict, and salivation occurs. *Nicotinic* receptors are found on skeletal muscle and autonomic ganglion cells. If these receptors are occupied by acetylcholine or a nicotinic drug, the muscles contract or the postganglionic neuron depolarizes. Acetylcholine will activate all cholinergic receptors and is rapidly inactivated by the enzyme, acetylcholinesterase. For these reasons, acetylcholine is *not employed as a drug*. Cholineric drugs are synthesized in laboratories and are made to specifically activate one type of receptor. Therefore, we have *nicotinic cholinergic drugs,* and we have *muscarinic cholinergic drugs.* Nicotinic drugs stimulate skeletal muscles and ganglia, while *muscarinic drugs* produce parasympathetic responses.[1]

Pilocarpine (Pilocar) and bethanechol (Urecholine) are the two most commonly employed *direct-acting* cholinergic drugs. While respectively used for their miotic (pupil constriction) and urinary effects, one should keep in mind that either drug is capable of producing any parasympathetic response as a side effect. While benefiting the patient with acute narrow angle glaucoma and urinary retention, either drug may produce bradycardia, bronchoconstriction, or salivation as side effects.

Indirect-acting cholinergic drugs do not function as agonists on cholinergic receptors. Instead, they act by inhibiting the enzyme, acetylcholinesterase, and therefore are commonly referred to as cholinesterase inhibitors, or anticholinesterase drugs. By inhibiting this enzyme, the body's acetylcholine is able to exert a prolonged effect on all cholinergic receptors.

> Cholinesterase inhibitors used in medicine produce their effect for a relatively brief time period. These drugs resemble acetylcholine in structure, generally not enough to compete for the cholinergic receptor, but enough to compete as a substrate for the enzyme, acetylcholinesterase. One should keep in mind that by inhibiting this enzyme, the effects produced by such a ubiquitous transmitter as acetylcholine may result in a staggering number of nicotinic and muscarinic responses. For this reason, when employing these drugs to promote cholinergic activity at skeletal muscle sites (myasthenia gravis) or at CNS locations (tranquilizer overdose), other drugs, such as atropine, may have to be utilized to block cholinergic side effects at muscarinic sites.[2]

While long-acting, irreversible inhibitors are employed in nerve gases and insecticides, the shorter-acting, reversible cholinesterase inhibitors are used for the same conditions as the direct-acting agents discussed above. Additionally, their cholinergic effect is lifesaving for patients suffering from myasthenia gravis. In this myopathy, cholinergic receptors on skeletal muscle are being destroyed by the patient's own immune system.[3] By increasing the levels of acetylcholine at these sites, muscle function returns. Table 3.1 lists some of the commonly employed cholinesterase inhibitors as well as direct-acting cholinergic agonists. Figure 3.1 illustrates the difference in mechanisms employed by cholinergic drugs.

TABLE 3.1 Commonly employed cholinergic agents

Cholinesterase Inhibitors	Direct-Acting
physostigmine (Antilirium)	pilocarpine (Pilocar)
neostigmine (Prostigmin)	bethanechol (Urecholine)
pyridostigmine (Mestinon)	carbachol (Isopto Carbachol)
edrophonium (Tensilon)	

Note: Trade names in parentheses follow the generic names.

Figure 3.1 Direct- and Indirect-Acting Cholinergic Drugs

A. Normal synaptic transmission occurs where acetylcholine (A) is released from the neurons and activates the receptor initiating a response. Acetylcholine is then destroyed by the enzyme acetylcholinesterase.

B. The direct-acting cholinergic drug (D) attaches to the receptor and initiates the response. Although acetylcholine (A) is not involved, it continues to be released by the neuronal ending and destroyed by acetylcholinesterase.

C. The cholinesterase inhibitor (X) is preventing the enzyme, acetylcholinesterase, from destroying acetylcholine (A). Therefore, the acetylcholine released by the neuronal ending accumulates and produces an exaggerated response by the organ.

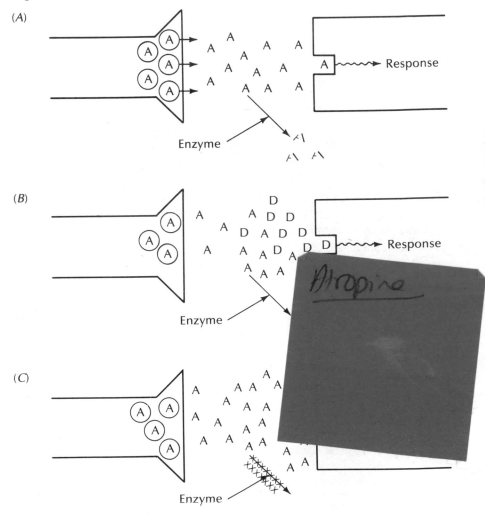

ANTICHOLINERGIC DRUGS

In Chapter 1 the receptor theory of drug action was presented. An agonist is a drug that occupies a receptor causing an effect, while antagonists competitively block this interaction. Anticholinergic drugs are classical examples of antagonists since they competitively block cholinergic receptors. In effect, they prevent acetylcholine and cholinergic drugs from activating their cholinergic receptors.

Atropine and Scopolamine are considered the prototypes of the anticholinergic drugs. You may want to picture their action as "permissive." By blocking acetylcholine's access to cholinergic receptors on cardiac and smooth-muscle cells, sympathetic innervation to these cells is permitted total dominance. It is therefore convenient, at least clinically, to view anticholinergic drugs as "permitting sympathetic effects" (see Figure 3.2).

Figure 3.2 Anticholinergic Mechanism
A. The heart rate is maintained at 72 due to a balance of parasympathetic and sympathetic innervation.
B. The anticholinergic drug (O) is blocking the cholinergic receptor, thus inhibiting acetylcholine's (A) ability to slow heart rate. This permits the sympathetic influence to dominate, thus increasing the heart rate.

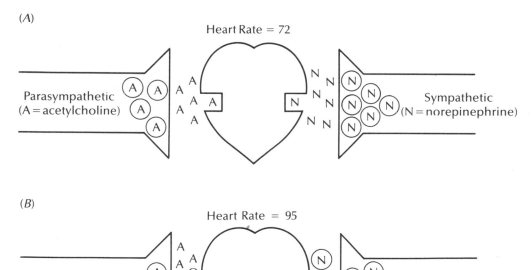

Following their administration, anticholinergic drugs inhibit alimentary and urinary motility, as well as salivary and respiratory tract secretions, and produce pupil dilatation. It is for this latter effect that the plant from which they were originally extracted was named belladonna (beautiful lady). It seems that long ago, women would rub the leaves of this plant in their eyes. The resulting mydriasis (pupil dilation) "weakened the hearts of their suitors."

Although anticholinergic drugs may produce an increased heart rate, they have no effect on the vascular system at therapeutic levels since, as stated earlier, the parasympathetic innervation to blood vessels is of little consequence.

> Cholinergic aspects of vascular control remain somewhat paradoxical. Following continuous intravenous infusion of acetylcholine or muscarinic agonists, vasodilation occurs, resulting in a significant drop in blood pressure. This seems evidence enough for the presence of cholinergic receptors on vascular smooth muscle. Contemporary thinking has acetylcholine being released from some of the sympathetic fibers which supply blood vessels, designating such fibers as "sympathetic cholinergics." Despite this confusion, most authorities agree that cholinergic phenomena associated with vascular control are physiologically and pharmacologically insignificant.[4]

Table 3.2 lists the more commonly employed anticholinergic drugs, and Table 3.3 lists common desired effects. Do not attempt to memorize these lists. Instead, study them as a lesson in logic. The "permissive" sympathetic effects produced by any anticholinergic drug, such as atropine, may be logically deduced by using the methods discussed in the previous chapter. Furthermore, one must realize that all the effects, other than the one for which the drug was indicated, must be considered secondary. For example, if atropine is administered to increase heart rate in the bradycardic patient, mydriasis and salivary inhibition must be considered side effects.

The use of cholinergic and anticholinergic agents in respiratory patients is somewhat limited but offers a good clinical example to conclude our discussion. Methacholine is a direct-acting cholinergic agonist employed as a diagnostic tool in asthmatic patients. Unlike bethanechol and pilocarpine, it is a substrate for acetylcholinesterase and therefore, is very brief in duration of action. During the so-called "methacholine challenge," patients inhale aerosolized solutions in varying concentrations. As you would expect, bronchoconstriction is the resultant effect and generally occurs with lower concentrations in asthmatic than in normal patients. An anticholinergic agent such as atropine should reverse the cholinergic effect of methacholine.[5]

TABLE 3.2   Commonly employed anticholinergic agents

hyoscine (Scopolamine)	dicyclomine (Bentyl)
atropine (Isopto Atropine)	glycopyrrolate (Robinul)
propantheline (Pro-Banthine)	tropicamide (Mydriacyl)

TABLE 3.3   Effects of anticholinergics*

Target Organ	Desired Effect
Eye	mydriasis
	cycloplegia
Heart	increased rate
	increased A-V conduction
GI	inhibit secretions
	decreased motility
	(antispasmodic)

*Most frequently, anticholinergics are employed for their effects on the eye, heart, and alimentary tract.

NEUROMUSCULAR BLOCKING AGENTS

Drugs that block the neurotransmission at skeletal muscle sites are conveniently classified according to their mechanism. *Competitive blockers* function purely as antagonists on these cholinergic receptors. Following receptor blockade, there are only limited numbers of receptors available for the acetylcholine released from the voluntary nerve fibers and depolarization of the muscle cell membrane cannot occur. D-tubocurarine, often called curare, remains the prototype of this class of blocker.

Agents such as succinylcholine (Anectine) produce their neuromuscular block in a distinctly different manner. These *depolarizing blockers* initially function as agonists on the receptor, thus initiating depolarization of the muscle membrane, as does acetylcholine. However, since succinylcholine is not a substrate for acetylcholinesterase, it persists on the receptor producing a repetitive excitatory effect on the muscle, witnessed clinically as transient muscular fasciculation. This phase passes quickly, and the drug remains on the receptor as an antagonist (blocker), much the same as d-tubocurarine (see Figure 3.3).

Figure 3.3

A. Acetylcholine is released from the voluntary fiber and attaches to the cholinergic
   receptor initiating depolarization of the muscle cell, following which, contraction
   will occur.

B. The competitive blocker, curare (c), occupies the receptor, thus limiting acetylcholine access. The muscle cannot depolarize.

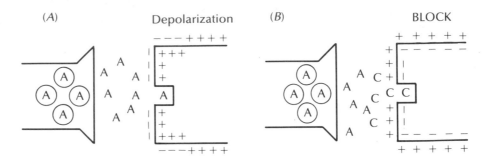

C. Succinylcholines initially depolarizes the muscle cell. Then the cell repolarizes
   with succinylcholine blocking acetylcholine's access to the receptor (much like
   curare did in B).

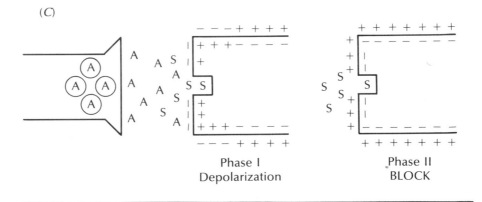

Both classes of muscle blockers are employed during surgery to facilitate
tracheal intubation and surgical manipulations. They may also be employed when
patients must be maintained on ventilators for extended time periods. Commonly
employed agents are listed in Table 3.4.

TABLE 3.4   Commonly employed neuromuscular blockers

Depolarizing Agents	Competitive Blockers
succinylcholine (Anectine)	d-tubocurarine (Tubarine)
decamethonium (Syncurine)	metocurine (Metubine)
	gallamine (Flaxedil)
	pancuronium (Pavulon)

Depolarizing agents such as succinylcholine are agonists with specific affinity for the nicotinic receptors on skeletal muscle membranes. Acetylcholine's effect on these receptors is brief (less than one second) owing to rapid hydrolysis by acetylcholinesterase. Because of this brevity, the skeletal muscle cell depolarizes, contracts, and repolarizes in preparation for the next contraction stimulus. Since it is not a substrate for acetylcholinesterase, succinylcholine remains on the receptor, producing repetitive depolarizations following which there ensues a competitive block. Succinylcholine's action is shorter than that of the "competitive blocker," usually ranging from three to five minutes. This is due to its hydrolysis by a plasma cholinesterase called pseudocholinesterase. Since the competitive blockers are quite lengthy in duration, they may be reversed by such cholinesterase inhibitors as prostigmine. In effect, the resulting levels of acetylcholine "overwhelm" and displace the competitive blockers from the receptors and initiate muscle depolarization and contraction.[6]

SYNOPSIS OF THERAPEUTIC AGENTS

I. Cholinergic drugs (direct-acting)

A. ACTION
   1. Function as agonists on cholinergic (muscarinic) receptors, thereby producing parasympathomimetic effects
B. COMMON INDICATIONS
   1. Glaucoma
   2. Urinary retention
C. PREPARATIONS
   1. Pilocarpine (Pilocar)
   2. Bethanechol (Urecholine)
D. SECONDARY EFFECTS
   1. Any undesired parasympathetic effect (To reader: practice deducing some of these)

II. Cholinergic drugs (indirect-acting)

A. ACTION
   1. Inhibit acetylcholinesterase, thereby potentiating the acetylcholine released by parasympathetic and voluntary motor nerves
B. COMMON INDICATIONS
   1. Glaucoma
   2. Myasthenia gravis
C. PREPARATIONS
   1. Physostigmine
D. SECONDARY EFFECTS
   1. Same as direct-acting cholinergic drugs

III. Anticholinergic agents

A. ACTION
   1. Function as antagonist on cholinergic (muscarinic) receptors, thereby producing effects the opposite of those produced by parasympathetic nerves
B. COMMON INDICATIONS (many uses)
   1. Preoperative medication
   2. Bradycardia
   3. Peptic ulcers
C. PREPARATIONS
   1. Atropine
D. SECONDARY EFFECTS
   1. Any undesired parasympatholytic effect (practice deducing some of these)

IV. Neuromuscular blocking agents

A. ACTION
1. Competitive blockers function as antagonists at cholinergic receptors on skeletal muscle cells
2. Depolarizing blockers initially stimulate the cholinergic receptors, following which they block the receptor similar to competitive blockers

B. COMMON INDICATIONS
1. Tracheal intubation during surgical procedures
2. Patients on ventilators

C. PREPARATIONS
1. Curare (competitive)
2. Succinylcholine (depolarizing)

ARTICLES FOR DISCUSSION

1. **Klock, L. E., et al.** 1975. A comparative study of atropine sulfate and isoproterenol hydrochloride in chronic bronchitis. *American Review of Respiratory Disease* 112:371–376.
2. **Di Palma, J. R.** 1974. Cholinergic and anticholinergic drugs. *RN* 37:83.
3. **Gal, T. S., and Suratt, P. M.** 1981. Atropine and glycopyrrolate effects on lung mechanics in normal man. *Anesthesia and Analgesia* 60:85–90.
4. **Stackhouse, J.** 1973. Myasthenia gravis. *American Journal of Nursing* 73:1544.
5. **Tinker, J. H., and Wehner, R. J.** 1974. Postoperative recovery and the neuromuscular junction. *American Journal of Nursing* 74:74.
6. **Abgelman, W., and Chodosh, S.** 1977. Bronchodilator action of the anticholinergic drug, ipratropium bromide (Sch 1000) as an aerosol in chronic bronchitis and asthma. *Chest* 71:324.
7. **Argov, Z., and Mastaglia, F. L.** 1979. Disorders of neuromuscular transmission caused by drugs. *New England Journal of Medicine* 301:409.
8. **Lee, C., and Katz, R. L.** 1980. Neuromuscular pharmacology: Clinical update and commentary. *British Journal of Anaesthesia* 52:173–188.

REFERENCES

1. Maze, M. 1981. Clinical implications of membrane receptor function in anesthesia. *Anesthesia* 55: 160–171.

2. Garber, J. G., et al. 1980. Physostigmine—atropine solution fails to reverse Diazepam sedation. *Anesthesia and Analgesia* 59: 58–60.

3. Isselbacher, K. J., et al. 1980. *Harrison's Principles of Internal Medicine,* 9th ed. New York: McGraw-Hill, 1980, pp. 2064–2067.

4. Goodman, L. S., and Gilman, A. 1980. *The Pharmacological Basis of Therapeutics.* 6th ed. New York: Macmillan, pp. 60–61.

5. Ziment, I. 1978. *Respiratory Pharmacology and Therapeutics.* Philadelphia: W. B. Saunders, pp. 437–439.

6. Goodman, L. S., and Gilman, A. 1980. *The Pharmacological Basis of Therapeutics.* 6th ed. New York: Macmillan, pp. 225–227.

4

Adrenergic Agonists and Antagonists

In the preceding chapter we centered our attention on drugs that block and imitate the effects of acetylcholine released by voluntary and parasympathetic nerves. It is now time to consider the actions of drugs that affect the sympathetic system. Any nerve that releases norepinephrine, epinephrine, or dopamine as its neurotransmitter is called an adrenergic nerve. Since this applies mainly to the postganglionic sympathetic neurons, the terms "sympathetic" and "adrenergic" may be used interchangeably. Any drug that imitates the actions of these sympathetic neurotransmitters is called an adrenergic drug. Those that block the action of these neurotransmitters are called adrenergic blockers.

ADRENERGIC RECEPTORS

You will recall that smooth, skeletal, and cardiac muscle cells contain receptors for acetylcholine, called cholinergic receptors. Smooth and cardiac muscle cells also contain receptors for adrenergic neurotransmitters that are appropriately called adrenergic receptors. (Naturally adrenergic receptors do not regulate skeletal muscle contraction since we have voluntary control over these cells.)

The adrenergic receptors are of three types, each producing a distinct response when activated by an appropriate agonist:

1. Alpha receptors produce smooth-muscle contraction.
2. Beta$_2$ receptors produce smooth-muscle relaxation.
3. Beta$_1$ receptors produce cardiac stimulation.

Generally speaking, each involuntary organ of the body is populated with only one primary type of adrenergic receptor. Adrenergic drugs are employed mainly for their effects on the bronchial muscle, pupils, and cardiovascular system. For this reason it may be convenient to memorize the typical distribution of receptors for these organs.

HEART: The primary receptor is beta$_1$ and when activated produces an increase in the rate and the force of contraction.

SUPERFICIAL ARTERIES: The primary receptor is alpha; when activated, it produces vasoconstriction.

VEINS AND DEEP ARTERIES: Both alpha and beta$_2$ receptors are present, thus providing a means for vasoconstriction or vasodilation depending on which receptor is stimulated.

BRONCHIOLES: The primary receptor is beta$_2$; when activated, it produces bronchodilation.

IRIS (RADIAL MUSCLE): The primary receptor is alpha; when activated, radial muscle contraction results in pupil dilatation (mydriasis).

Keep in mind that, with the exception of blood vessels, the opposite effects from those described above are produced by parasympathetic innervation. While beta$_2$ receptors provide sympathetic-mediated bronchodilation, cholinergic receptors (not alpha receptors) provide parasympathetic-mediated bronchoconstriction.

Although each involuntary organ contains a mixture of the three adrenergic receptor types, it is generally accepted that one receptor is overwhelmingly predominant. While the heart is easily remembered as possessing only beta$_1$ receptors, our concern is to establish whether alpha or beta$_2$ receptors are predominant in each of the remaining organs. Although Table 4.1 illustrates the receptor locations and autonomic control of body organs, memorization of such a list is, at the very least, discouraging. To logically deduce the predominant receptor, establish the sympathetic effect on the organ using the format described in Chapter 2. Once you have established this, the receptor type will be obvious when you consider that alpha receptors constrict while beta$_2$ receptors relax. For example, if you deduce that inhibition or relaxation of the urinary bladder is appropriate during fight or flight, it should follow that beta$_2$ is the predominant adrenergic receptor found in the urinary bladder and mediates sympathetic relaxation. It would also follow that parasympathetic nerves produce bladder contraction through cholinergic receptor activation.

TABLE 4.1 Autonomic control of body organs

Organ	Receptor	Sympathetic Response	Parasympathetic Response
Iris			
radial muscle	alpha	contraction (mydriasis)	none
sphincter	none	none	contraction (miosis)
Heart	$beta_1$	increase rate, contractility, and neuroconduction	decrease rate, contractility, and neuroconduction
Arteries			
skin and mucosa	alpha	constriction	insignificant
others	alpha, $beta_2$	constriction or dilation	insignificant
Veins	alpha, $beta_2$	constriction or dilation	insignificant
Lung			
bronchial muscle	$beta_2$	relaxation	contraction
secretions		insignificant	stimulation
Salivary and nasopharyngeal		insignificant	stimulation of secretion
GI Tract			
motility	$beta_2$	decrease	increase relaxation,
sphincters	alpha	contraction	stimulation
secretion		insignificant	
Kidney	$beta_2$	renin secretion	none
Bladder			
detrusor	$beta_2$	relaxation	contraction
sphincter	alpha	contraction	relaxation
Male Sex Organs	alpha	ejaculation	erection

Modified from Goodman, L. S., and Gilman, A. 1980. *The Pharmacological Basis of Therapeutics*, 6th ed., New York, Macmillan.

Innervation to sweat glands offers a curious exception to the logic of autonomic control since postganglionic sympathetic fibers to these glands release acetylcholine instead of norepinephrine. Therefore, even though sweating is a sympathetic effect, its mechanism is cholinergic and is therefore stimulated by cholinergic agonists and inhibited by anticholinergic agents. As an example, the phenomenon referred to as "atropine flush" occurs following the administration of high doses of anticholinergic agents. It is believed that vasodilation of cutaneous vessels may occur in order to provide a means of heat loss following the inhibition of sweating, the usual mechanism for heat loss.[1]

CHEMICAL NATURE OF ADRENERGIC NEUROTRANSMITTERS

Adrenergic neurotransmitters are endogenously produced chemicals having a catechol group linked to an ethylamine group:

$$\text{HO} - \bigcirc - \text{HO} \quad | \quad CH_2 - CH_2 - NH_2 \quad |$$

Catechol   Ethylamine
Group   Group

For this reason, these neurotransmitters are sometimes referred to as *catecholamines*. Their synthesis takes place in adrenergic nerve terminals and in the adrenal medulla beginning with the familiar amino acid, tyrosine (see Figure 4.1). While the exact chemical changes are not essential to memorize, the sequence of conversion from dopa to dopamine to norepinephrine to epinephrine has several clinical applications. For example, Parkinson's disease is generally considered to result from a deficiency of dopamine in the basal ganglia. It would seem logical to administer dopamine to these patients. However, dopamine, as well as other catecholamines, has very poor lipid solubility and fails to penetrate the blood-brain barrier. Interestingly enough, dopa, the immediate synthetic precursor to dopamine, is actively transported through this "barrier" and penetrates the basal ganglia where it is converted to dopamine. This discovery has provided a major breakthrough in the treatment of patients suffering Parkinson's disease.

In the last chapter we learned that the parasympathetic neurotransmitter, acetylcholine, was terminated by an enzyme called *acetylcholinesterase* (AChE). As explained in Chapter 2, the effects of catecholamine neurotransmitters are terminated in three ways:

1. An enzyme called monoamine oxidase (MAO) alters the amine group, rendering the chemical inactive.
2. An enzyme called catechol-o-methyltransferase (COMT) transfers a methyl group to the catechol complex, which renders the chemical inactive.
3. However, the most significant termination is by the nerve ending's ability to take up the released neurotransmitter and eventually use it again.

Figure 4.1

Synthetic pathway for catecholamines. The modification from the immediate precursor is circled.

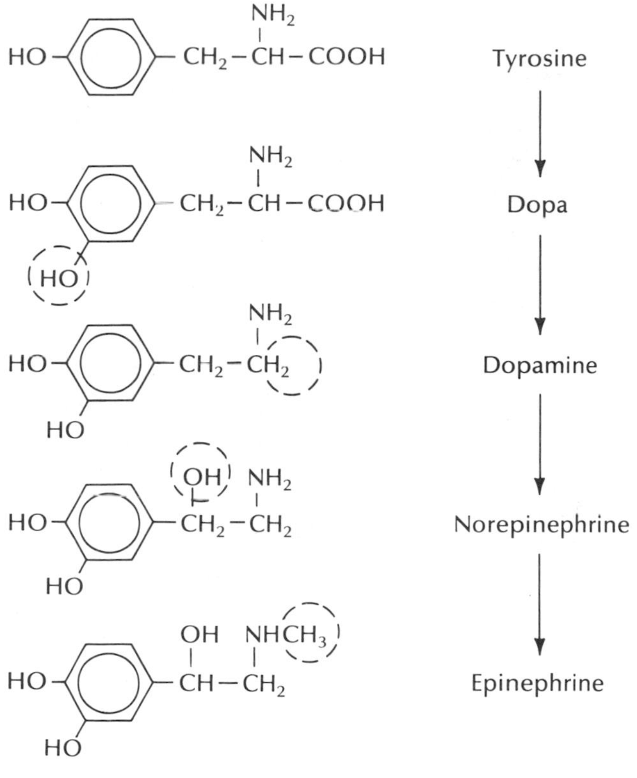

ADRENERGIC DRUGS

Drugs synthesized to activate the adrenergic receptors vary in their chemical structure. Some have the catecholamine arrangement, but others lack the exact catechol structure and therefore cannot be classified as catecholamines even though they all contain an amine group. As an example, compare isoproterenol hydrochloride (Isuprel) with terbutaline sulfate (Brethine):

HO —⬡— CH—CH—NH   (Isoproterenol)
HO | | |
          OH H CH(CH₃)₂

HO
⬡— CH—CH—NH   (Terbutaline)
          | | |
          OH H   C(CH₃)₃
HO

Notice that, while similar in structure, terbutaline does not contain the catechol group. Since some adrenergic drugs are not catechols, but *all* contain amine groupings, we commonly refer to all adrenergic drugs as being *"sympathomimetic amines."* The major clinical significance of this structural issue is the fact that noncatecholamines have a longer duration of action because they avoid biotransformation by the specific enzyme, catechol-o-methyl transferase (COMT).

Adrenergic drugs and neurotransmitters are characterized according to their ability to activate alpha or beta receptors. If you know the predominant receptor in an organ, you can then predict the effect of the drug in question. For example, phenylephrine (Neo-Synephrine) is an alpha-adrenergic drug. It will constrict blood vessels since they contain alpha receptors, but will have no direct effect on the heart since it contains beta₁ receptors.

It is possible to deduce logically a drug's effect on any organ by knowing only its receptor affinity—even without knowing the type of receptor in the organ. Let us test our ability to reason: Isoproterenol is a beta₁- and beta₂-adrenergic agonist. What will be its effect on bronchial muscle? Try the following line of reasoning:

1. When we say adrenergic, we are dealing with sympathetic responses.
2. What must the bronchioles do during times of fight or flight?
   Answer: They must dilate.
3. Is smooth muscle relaxation characteristic of alpha or beta₁ or beta₂ receptors?
   Answer: Beta₂ receptors cause smooth muscle relaxation.
4. Does the drug in question have beta₂ properties?
   Answer: Yes.
5. Isoproterenol will dilate the bronchial passages.

What effect would an alpha-adrenergic drug, such as Neo-Synephrine, have on the bronchial smooth muscle? After going through the above reasoning steps, you should come up with the answer, "No effect," since you have established that bronchial smooth muscle contains only beta$_2$ receptors.

Adrenergic drugs offer an excellent example of "structural-activity relationships." This concept deals with the relationship between the molecular structural arrangement of a drug and its affinity for specific receptor types. For example, all adrenergic drugs are comprised of a phenyl ring with an ethylamine side chain. Substitutions of hydroxyl groups on the phenyl ring and alkyl groups on the nitrogen atom determine the drug's affinity for either alpha, beta$_1$, or beta$_2$ receptors. Notice in the following examples how dihydroxyl substitutions and alkyl substitutions confer beta receptor specificity.

OH
|
⬡—CH—CH$_2$—NH
＼CH$_3$ Phenylephrine (alpha)

OH
|
HO—⬡—CH—CH$_2$—NH$_2$ Norepinephrine (alpha, beta,)
HO

OH
|
HO—⬡—CH—CH$_2$—NH
＼CH$_3$ Epinephrine (alpha, beta$_1$, beta$_2$)
HO

OH
|
HO—⬡—CH—CH$_2$—NH
CH(CH$_3$)$_2$ Isoproterenol (beta$_1$, beta$_2$)
HO

Although quite complex, this intriguing concept provides a basis for pharmacologists to develop drugs that are more specific in action thereby limiting undesirable side effects. For example, the slight structural difference between isoproterenol and terbutaline (see above) lessens the beta$_1$ cardiotonic actions of terbutaline to such an extent that it is generally recognized as the most specific beta$_2$-adrenergic drug available.

Indirect-Acting Adrenergic Drugs

From our discussion thus far, it would seem that all adrenergic drugs are agonists for adrenergic receptors and are, therefore, *direct-acting*. This is not always the case. Many adrenergic drugs have an indirect mechanism of action. These drugs actually stimulate the adrenergic nerve endings to release norepinephrine. Therefore it is actually the patient's own norepinephrine that produces the sympathetic response. Such drugs as metaraminol (Aramine) and the various amphetamines utilize this mechanism of action.

Further complicating this issue is the fact that some drugs have a dual mechanism of action, in that they function as agonists on adrenergic receptors and also stimulate the release of norepinephrine. The most popular mixed-action adrenergic drug is ephedrine.

Therapeutic Uses of Adrenergic Drugs

The more commonly employed adrenergic drugs are listed in Table 4.2. Adrenergic drugs are commonly employed to treat upper respiratory congestion. Congestion of upper respiratory passages is actually a swelling of mucosa and is a result of vasodilation of mucosal arteries. Obviously decongestion is accomplished by constricting these vessels. Since alpha receptors are responsible for constricting blood vessels, an alpha-adrenergic drug such as Neo-Synephrine is the popular therapeutic choice. Rebound congestion is an interesting side effect that occurs following frequent use of decongestants. In this phenomenon, shortly after the administration of a nasal spray, the nasal mucosa swells greater than before, thus requiring the individual to use the drug with even greater frequency. It is common for patients experiencing this phenomenon to claim they are "hooked" on the medication.

TABLE 4.2 Commonly used adrenergic drugs

Name	Receptor Affinity
epinephrine (Adrenalin)	alpha, beta$_1$, beta$_2$
norepinephrine (Levophed)	alpha, beta$_1$
isoproterenol (Isuprel)	beta$_1$, beta$_2$
isoetharine (Bronkosol)	beta$_2$
terbutaline (Brethine)	beta$_2$
dobutamine (Dobutrex)	beta$_1$
dopamine (Intropin)	alpha, beta$_1$, beta$_2$, dopaminergic
phenylephrine (Neo-Synephrine)	alpha
ritodrine (Yuptopar)	beta$_2$

Rebound congestion offers a good example of altered receptor population. Frequent activation of adrenergic receptors has been shown to result in a reduction in the number of receptor sites.[2] In the above example, frequent use of alpha agonists results in a reduction of alpha receptors in the nasal mucosa. This, coupled with the inflammatory potential of nasal sprays, results in severe congestion refractory to decongestant therapy.

This same concept is found in asthmatics who are overzealous in their use of beta-adrenergic inhalants. The resulting decrease in beta-receptor population accounts for the frequency of bronchospastic episodes and refractoriness to treatment. It is interesting to note that an opposite effect on receptor number occurs when receptors are not utilized for prolonged periods. Patients taking beta-receptor–blocking drugs have been shown to develop an increased beta-receptor population. Upon abrupt withdrawal of the medication, beta organs, such as the heart, are overly sensitive to stimulation by the beta-adrenergic agonist.[3]

In patients with asthma or other forms of bronchospasm, the bronchial smooth muscle must be relaxed so the bronchioles can dilate. The adrenergic receptor here is $beta_2$ thus indicating beta-adrenergic drugs, such as epinephrine or isoproterenol, as the drugs of choice. It is important to remember that since both of these drugs possess $beta_1$ as well as $beta_2$ properties, cardiac stimulation may be a serious side effect. Isoetharine (Bronkosol) is often used in respiratory therapy because of its selective $beta_2$ receptor affinity (see Table 4.2).

In anaphylactic shock there are two conditions that threaten the life of a patient. Extensive vasodilation produces severe hypotension and laryngeal edema, while bronchospasm threatens respiratory exchange. In treating this dramatic emergency, a drug with vessel-constricting ability and bronchial relaxation capabilities is necessary. Epinephrine, which possesses both alpha and beta properties, is the universal drug of choice for correcting this life-threatening condition.

In cardiac arrest, due either to ventricular fibrillation or asystole, a drug with strong $beta_1$ activity is indicated. Epinephrine is generally the drug recommended by emergency-room physicians in this situation.

The treatment of hypotension and shock presents an interesting dilemma in selecting adrenergic drugs. It always seemed logical to attempt correction of hypotensive episodes by administering alpha-adrenergic drugs which, obviously, constrict blood vessels thus elevating blood pressure. Unfortunately vasoconstriction increases the effort of the heart to pump blood through these narrowed arteries (afterload), and constriction of renal arteries may seriously impair renal perfusion and thus glomerular filtration.[4] These problems create a unique place for the use of dopamine (Intropin), especially in cardiogenic shock. Not only does dopamine stimulate alpha and beta receptors, but it also has a unique affinity for specialized dilating receptors in the renal arteries appropriately called dopaminergic receptors. Thus we have a drug that, while constricting most blood vessels, also stimulates the heart and dilates the renal arteries, thus assuring adequate renal perfusion.

> Dopamine offers a complex but interesting lesson in adrenergic receptor affinity. At low-dosage infusion rates (2 to 5 mcg/kg/min), affinity for dopaminergic receptors dominates. As dosage is increased, the affinity for beta and then alpha receptors becomes apparent until, at high doses, dopamine's alpha-receptor activity may be so dominant as to override dopaminergic-receptor function. This will result in the same renal shutdown seen with pure alpha-adrenergic drugs. For this reason, patients infused with dopamine must be continuously monitored for heart rate, blood pressure, and urine output.[5]

> Indeed, this variation in receptor affinity is seen with other agents possessing mixed-receptor affinity. In very low doses, epinephrine has a stronger affinity for beta receptors than alpha receptors. Therefore tachycardia, and beta$_2$-receptor–mediated vasodilation may occur, producing a seemingly paradoxical drop in blood pressure. However, the usual therapeutic doses are high enough to activate both alpha and beta$_2$ receptors, in which case, alpha-induced vasoconstriction dominates.[6]

ADRENERGIC BLOCKERS

In Chapter 3, it was stated that there are specific antagonist drugs which block the agonist, acetylcholine, from attaching to cholinergic receptors. We also have antagonist drugs for each adrenergic receptor that will block this receptor from adrenergic agonists. The most commonly employed drugs of this class are phentolamine (Regitine), which blocks alpha receptors, and propranolol (Inderal), which blocks beta receptors.

By blocking norepinephrine's access to alpha receptors, phentolamine (Regitine) produces a vasodilation that may be useful in treating certain types of hypertensive crisis. Another interesting use of Regitine is during Levophed infusions. Levophed is a brand of norepinephrine that may be continuously infused during hypotensive episodes. It is a very potent and efficacious vasoconstrictor and, should the infusion extravasate, subcutaneous blood vessels in the venipuncture area will constrict so severely that local ischemia will result in tissue necrosis and sloughing. Low doses of Regitine, infused simultaneously with this Levophed drip, will counteract this severe vasoconstriction should extravasation occur.

Propranolol is used clinically for its ability to block the beta$_1$ receptors of the heart. In essence, this removes sympathetic influence on the heart and permits parasympathetic predomination to slow the heart's activity. This proves useful in treating certain dysrythmias, hypertension, and angina pectoris. The major drawback of propranolol is that it also blocks beta$_2$ receptors, which may permit cholinergic-induced bronchospasm. Newer beta blockers, such as metoprolol (Lopressor), are reported to have relative specificity for only beta$_1$ receptors, and therefore may be preferred in asthmatic patients. The increasing number of beta blockers being introduced certainly witnesses the effectiveness of this drug class (see Table 4.3). Recent evidence supporting their effectiveness in preventing recurrences of myocardial infarction adds another indication to an already impressive list of indications for beta adrenoreceptor blockers.

TABLE 4.3   Beta-adrenergic blockers

Beta$_1$ and beta$_2$ blockers (nonselective)	Beta$_1$ blockers (cardioselective)
propranolol (Inderal)	metoprolol (Lopressor)
nadolol (Corgard)	atenolol (Tenormin)
timolol (Blocadren)	

The effect of beta blockers on skeletal muscle bloodflow during strenuous activity is presently receiving considerable attention. It would seem that beta-receptor blockade on skeletal muscle arteries would compromise bloodflow. During strenuous activity, the epinephrine released by the adrenal medulla should have a greater effect on the available alpha receptors, thus stimulating vasoconstriction and diminishing bloodflow. If this is true, athletic patients requiring beta-blocker therapy should fare better if treated with specific beta$_1$ blockers such as metoprolol (Lopressor). However, at the present time studies conflict on this issue.[7, 8]

SYNOPSIS OF THERAPEUTIC AGENTS

I. Adrenergic agents

A. ACTION
   1. Function as agonists on alpha and/or beta receptors, thereby producing sympathomimetic effects

B. COMMON INDICATIONS
   1. Alpha agonists
      a) Hypotension
      b) Opthalmic examination (mydriasis)
      c) Reduce hemorrhage during surgical procedures
   2. Beta agonists
      a) Cardiac arrest
      b) Bronchospasm
   3. Combined alpha and beta agonists
      a) All of above
      b) Anaphylactic shock

C. PREPARATIONS
   1. Alpha agonists
      a) Phenylephrine (Neo-Synephrine)
   2. Beta agonists
      a) Isoproterenol (Isuprel)
   3. Combined
      a) Epinephrine (Adrenalin)
      b) Dopamine (Intropin)

D. SECONDARY EFFECTS
   1. Any undesired sypathomimetic effects (To reader: practice deducing these)

II. Adrenergic blockers

A. ACTION
   1. Function as antagonist on either alpha or beta receptors, thus preventing the normal sympathetic effect

B. COMMON INDICATIONS
   1. Beta blockers
      a) Angina
      b) Hypertension
      c) Cardiac dysrythmias
   2. Alpha blockers
      a) Hypertension

II. Adrenergic blockers (*continued*)

  C. PREPARATIONS
    1. Beta blocker
      a) Propranolol (Inderal)
    2. Alpha blocker
      a) Phentolamine (Regitine)
  D. SECONDARY EFFECTS
    1. Beta blockers
      a) Bradycardia
      b) Bronchospasm
    2. Alpha blockers
      a) Miosis
      b) Hypotension

ARTICLES FOR DISCUSSION

1. **Kelly, J. F., et al.** 1974. Anaphylaxis: Course, mechanisms, and treatment. *JAMA* 227:1431–1436.
2. **Murren, O.** 1980. New drugs in the treatment of bronchial asthma. *Hospital Formulary* 15:363.
3. **Nordstrom, L. A.** 1975. Effect of propranolol on respiratory function and exercise tolerance in patients with chronic obstructive lung disease. *Chest* 67:287.
4. **Leifer, K. N., and Witlig, H. J.** 1975. The beta-2 sympathomimetic aerosols in the treatment of asthma. *Annals of Allergy* 35:69.
5. **Tolas, A. G., et al.** 1982. Arterial plasma epinephrine concentrations and hemodynamic responses after dental injection of local anesthesia with epinephrine. *Journal of the American Dental Association* 104:41.
6. **Wiley, L.** 1974. Shock. II. Different kinds—different problems. *Nursing 74* 4:43.
7. **Moyer, J. H., and Mills, L. C.** 1975. Vasopressor agents in shock. *American Journal of Nursing* 75:620–625.
8. **Sklar, J., et al.** 1982. The effects of a cardioselective (metoprolol) and nonselective (propranolol) beta-adrenergic blocker on the response to dynamic exercise in normal man. *Circulation* 65:894–899.
9. **Smith, R. S., and Warren, D. J.** 1982. Effect of beta blocking drugs on peripheral blood flow in intermittent claudication. *Journal of Cardiovascular Pharmacology* 4:2–4.

REFERENCES

1. **Goodman, L. S., and Gilman, A.** 1980. *The Pharmacological Basis of Therapeutics*, 6th ed. New York: Macmillan.

2. **Motulsky, J. J., and Insel, P. A.** 1982. Adrenergic receptors in man: Direct identification, physiologic regulation, and clinical alterations. *New England Journal of Medicine* 307:18–29.

3. **Aarons, R. D., et al.** 1980. Elevation of b-adrenergic receptor density in human lymphocytes after propranolol administration. *Journal of Clinical Investigation* 65:949–957.

4. **Tarazi, R. C.** 1974. Sympathomimetic agents in the treatment of shock. *Annals of Internal Medicine* 81:364–371.

5. **McIntyre, K. M., and Lewis, A. J.,** eds. 1981. *Textbook of Advanced Cardiac Life Support,* American Heart Association. Dallas, Texas.

6. **Bhagat, B. D.** 1979. *Mode of Action of Autonomic Drugs.* Graceway Publishing Company. Flushing, New York.

7. **McSorley, P. D., and Warren, D. S.** 1978. Effects of propranolol and metoprolol on the peripheral circulation. *British Medical Journal* 3:1598.

8. **Sklar, J., et al.** 1982. The effects of a cardioselective (metoprolol) and a nonselective (propranolol) beta-adrenergic blocker on the response to dynamic exercise in normal men. *Circulation* 65:894–899.

5

Local Anesthetics

In Chapter 2 we learned that a nerve impulse is actually neuronal membrane de-polarization that results from the influx of sodium ions. When a local anesthetic is placed in the proximity of a nerve, the drug blocks the membrane sodium chan-nels. Thus the cell remains impermeable to sodium, even when stimulated. In this manner, nerve impulse transmission is prevented (see Figure 5.1). Although im-pulses in both motor and sensory nerves may be inhibited, the clinical use of local anesthetics is intended to block sensory impulses from reaching the central ner-vous system. However, if deposited near mixed-nerve trunks, it is not uncommon for motor impulse blockade to occur resulting in a temporary loss of voluntary and/or autonomic motor function.

Figure 5.1   Mechanism of Local Anesthetic Block

A. Normally, following a stimulus, the neural membrane becomes permeable to so-dium and sodium diffuses inward through sodium channels.

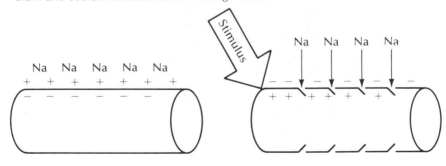

B. If local anesthetic ⒧Ⓐ is deposited in the vicinity of the neuron, the sodium channels are blocked by the anesthetic, thus preventing the inward sodium flow. In this case, depolarization of the neu-ronal membrane cannot proceed.

Sensory and motor neurons vary extensively in terms of diameter and myelination and therefore in what is termed "critical length." While far too complex for our present discussion, it is enough to say that there *does* exist a "preferential susceptibility" among neuronal fibers for local anesthetic blockade. In a mixed-nerve trunk, pain fibers are more susceptible to local anesthetics than pressure fibers or various motor fibers. For this reason, local anesthetic infiltrations generally produce a sensory loss without interrupting normal efferent neural functions.[1]

AVAILABLE PREPARATIONS

Local anesthetics are conveniently divided into two classes—the esters and the amides. Procaine (Novocain) is the most familiar of the esters, a group that has been essentially retired in favor of the amides. Members of the amide group have proven less toxic, as well as more efficacious, and presently dominate the therapeutic market. While lidocaine (Xylocaine) remains the most heralded member of this group, amides with greater potency and duration are gaining in popularity. Table 5.1 lists the more commonly employed local anesthetics.

TABLE 5.1 Commonly used local anesthetics

Ester Derivatives	*Amide Derivatives*
procaine (Novocain)	*lidocaine (Xylocaine)
chloroprocaine (Nesacaine)	mepivacaine (Carbocaine)
*benzocaine (Hurricaine)	prilocaine (Citanest)
*tetracaine (Pontocaine)	bupivacaine (Marcaine)
	etidocaine (Duranest)

*Useful as topical agents

All local anesthetics, both esters and amides, share three similar structural components (see Table 5.2):

1. Fat-soluble (lipophilic) aromatic ring.
2. Intermediate chain (either ester or amide).
3. Water-soluble (hydrophilic) amino terminal group.

It is usually accepted that both lipophilic and hydrophilic portions are required for effective blockade of sodium channels in the neuronal membrane. The lipophilic portion facilitates diffusion into the lipid portion of the membrane while the hydrophilic portion, and perhaps the lipophilic portion, block the sodium channels.[2]

Table 5.2   Structural formulas of commonly employed local anesthetics

Aromatic residue	Intermediate chain	Amino terminus	Aromatic residue	Intermediate chain	Amino terminus
	ESTERS		CH_3	AMIDES	
H_2N—⟨○⟩—	$COOCH_2CH_2$—	$N \begin{smallmatrix} C_2H_3 \\ C_2H_3 \end{smallmatrix}$	⟨○⟩— CH_3	$NHCOCH_2$—N	$\begin{smallmatrix} C_2H_3 \\ C_2H_3 \end{smallmatrix}$
	Procaine			Lidocaine	
$\begin{smallmatrix} H_3C_2 \\ N \\ H \end{smallmatrix}$ —⟨○⟩—	$COOCH_2CH_2$—N	$\begin{smallmatrix} CH_3 \\ CH_3 \end{smallmatrix}$	⟨○⟩ $\begin{smallmatrix} CH_3 \\ CH_3 \end{smallmatrix}$	$NHCOCH$—N	C_3H_2
	Tetracaine			Mepivacaine	
H_2N—⟨○⟩—	$COOCH_2CH_3$		⟨○⟩ $\begin{smallmatrix} CH_3 \\ CH_3 \end{smallmatrix}$	$NHCOCH$—N $\begin{smallmatrix} CH_3 \\ \end{smallmatrix}$	$\begin{smallmatrix} H \\ C_2H_3 \end{smallmatrix}$
	Benzocaine			Prilocaine	

From Neidle, E. A., et al. 1980. *Pharmacology and Therapeutics for Dentistry*. St. Louis: C. V. Mosby.

ADVERSE REACTIONS

Although adverse reactions have been documented, they are surprisingly infrequent. Convulsions, following systemic absorption of high doses, are the most serious consequence.

> The exact mechanism whereby local anesthetics produce seizure activity within the CNS remains confusing. This is especially true in light of the fact that lidocaine may actually be useful in depressing certain seizure disorders. Present theories center around the drug's dose-related affinity for either the inhibitory or excitatory tracts composing the reticular activating system. Toxic doses are thought to depress impulse conduction through the inhibitory tracts, thus potentiating the cerebral effects of the unopposed excitatory tracts.[3]

Relatively few cases of hypersensitivity have been documented and, when established, have generally been attributed to a common preservative, methylparaben, rather than to the local anesthetic itself.[4] If a true allergy exists to one of the ester-type anesthetics, an amide derivative can be safely employed. It is also worth noting that there does not seem to be any cross-hypersensitivity between local anesthetics within the amide group.

USE OF VASOCONSTRICTORS

Except for the administration of spinal anesthetics, most local anesthetics are administered as subcutaneous infiltrations for field or nerve trunk blocks. As you will see, it is an advantage to keep the anesthetic confined to the area in which it is injected. Since absorption into the surrounding blood vessels offers the major threat of transporting the anesthetic to undesirable regions, constricting these vessels limits this possibility. We have learned that alpha-adrenergic drugs constrict blood vessels, and therefore they are added to local anesthetics. This results in three therapeutic advantages by delaying absorption from the injection site:

1. Increased depth and duration of anesthesia.
2. Decreased systemic toxicity.
3. Due to vasoconstriction, the area of an injection is less hemorrhagic.

It is essential to consider this vasoconstricting action when operating on areas of the body having poor collateral circulation, such as the penis, superficial skin, fingers, and ears. In these areas, indiscriminate use of local anesthetics containing vasoconstrictors may result in severe ischemia resulting in necrosis and tissue sloughing. The most commonly employed vasoconstrictors are epinephrine and levonordefrin (Neo-Cobefrin).

There is often a controversy over the significance of using epinephrine with local anesthetics in patients suffering various forms of cardiovascular disease. One need only consider the small amount of epinephrine used and its great advantage in preventing local anesthetic absorption to dispel this concern. Most local anesthetics contain an epinephrine concentration of 1:100,000. This converts to .01 mg per ml or .04 mg of subcutaneously administered epinephrine for a 4 cc infiltration of local anesthetic. This becomes even more insignificant when one considers epinephrine's short duration of action due to neuronal uptake, biotransformation by COMT, and to a lesser extent, MAO. The adrenal medulla of a resting adult who weighs 70 kg secretes approximately .002 mg of epinephrine and norepinephrine each minute.[5] When one considers that this represents an intravenous infusion and may increase drastically should adequate anesthesia not be obtained, it is not surprising that the New York Heart Association does not object to doses of epinephrine up to .2 mg in patients with heart disease.[6, 7]

CLINICAL USES OF LOCAL ANESTHETICS

Lidocaine is probably the most widely used local anesthetic. In the next module, we will discuss its use in treating cardiac arrhythmias, but for now, we will only discuss its use for anesthetic purposes.

Although most patients refer to all local anesthetics as "Novocain," lidocaine is the most widely used anesthetic in all areas of health care. Topical sprays are employed to anesthetize the upper respiratory passages for procedures such as endotracheal intubation, bronchoscopy, and minor surgical procedures. Lidocaine, with epinephrine, is the most common agent employed by dentists, although mepivacaine has grown in popularity. Lidocaine is still a favorite among anesthesiologists for spinal anesthesia. It is interesting to note that the lidocaine is often mixed with 10 percent glucose to add weight to the solution. This hyperbaric solution prevents the lidocaine from diffusing to higher levels of the cord where the anesthesia may interfere with respiratory and cardiovascular functions.

It is not uncommon for patients to complain of adverse reactions to "Novocain." Understanding the various reactions possible will prevent this complaint from being misconstrued as an allergic reaction. The following represent the more common reactions experienced:

1. Psychogenic syncope is a common form of fainting patients may experience when receiving *any* injection, especially intraoral.
2. Local anesthetics containing epinephrine may produce palpitations or a transient tachycardia from the beta-adrenergic activity of epinephrine. Levonordefrin (Neo-Cobefrin), contained in mepivacaine preparations, is less likely to cause this effect.
3. Although allergies are possible, they are rare with the amide group of local anesthetics. Recall that if true hypersensitivity symptoms do occur, they are more likely to be associated with ester derivatives or the preservative called methylparaben.

SYNOPSIS OF THERAPEUTIC AGENTS

I. Local anesthetics

A. ACTION
1. Block inward flow of sodium ions, thereby preventing the transmission of neural impulses
B. COMMON INDICATIONS
1. Anesthesia for surgical procedures
2. Cardiac dysrhythmias
C. PREPARATION
1. Lidocaine (Xylocaine)
D. SECONDARY EFFECTS
1. Paresthesia
2. Myocardial depression
3. Convulsive seizures

ARTICLES FOR DISCUSSION

1. **Cannel H., et al.** 1975. Circulating levels of lignocaine after perioral injections. *British Dental Journal* 138:87–93.
2. **Miller, W. C., and Awe, R.** 1975. Effect of nebulized Lidocaine on reactive airways. *American Review of Respiratory Disease* 111:739–741.
3. **Wilbur, H. O., and Ovelette, T. R.** 1976. Topical anesthesia to improve patient tolerance of artificial airways during mechanical ventilation. *Respiratory Care* 21:617–619.
4. **Chu, S. S., et al.** 1975. Plasma concentration of lidocaine after endotracheal spray. *Anesthesia and Analgesia* 54:438–441.
5. **Brown, W. V., et al.** 1975. Newborn blood levels of lidocaine and mepivacaine in the first postnatal day following maternal epidural anesthesia. *Anesthesiology* 42:698.
6. **Nocolls, E. T., et al.** 1981. Epidural anesthesia for the woman in labor. *American Journal of Nursing* 81:1826–1830.
7. **Rothstein P., et al.** 1982. Prolonged seizures associated with the use of viscous lidocaine. *Journal of Pediatrics* 101:461–463.

REFERENCES

1. **Gissen, A. J., et al.** 1980. Differential sensitivities of mammalian nerve fibers to local anesthetic agents. *Anesthesiology* 53:467–474.

2. **Justak, J. T., and Yagiela, J. A.** 1981. *Regional Anesthesia of the Oral Cavity.* St. Louis: C. V. Mosby, p. 38.

3. **Covino, B. G.** 1972. Local anesthesia. *New England Journal of Medicine* 286:975 (Part I), 1035 (Part II).

4. **Luebke, N. H., and Walker, J. A.** 1978. Discussion of sensitivity to preservatives in anesthetics. *Journal of the American Dental Association* 97:656–657.

5. **Guyton, A. C.** 1981. *Textbook of Medical Physiology,* 6th ed. Philadelphia: W. B. Saunders.

6. **Committee Report.** 1964. Management of dental problems in patients with cardiovascular diseases. *Journal of the American Dental Association* 68:333.

7. **Committee Report.** 1955. Use of epinephrine in connection with procaine in dental procedures. *Journal of the American Dental Association* 50:108.

6

Cardiovascular Function

The cardiovascular system consists of a muscular pump that is primed by venous return of blood and subsequently ejects its contents into arteries. The entire system is lined with a layer of endothelium referred to as endocardium in the heart and intima in the vessels. The major portion of the system also contains a muscular layer most prominent in the heart (myocardium) and great arteries (media), less prominent in the great veins, and absent in the capillaries and the venules.

Figure 6.1
The direction of flow may be easier to appreciate if we modify the actual circulation patterns shown in Figure 6.2.

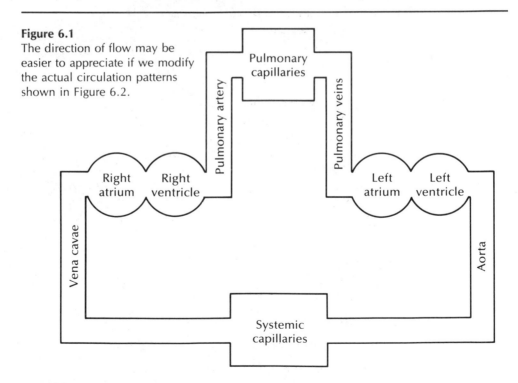

By studying the diagrams in Figures 6.1 and 6.2, you may review major anatomical components as well as the direction of flow.

Figure 6.2   Pulmonary and Systemic Circulation Patterns

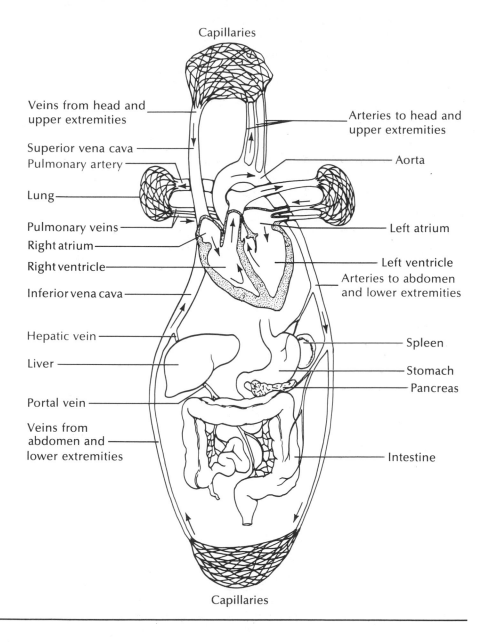

THE CARDIAC CYCLE

Before the ventricles contract (systole), they must be filled with blood returning from the venae cavae and the pulmonary veins. This filling volume is referred to as end-diastolic volume or *preload*. Most of the preload (70 percent) occurs passively while the atria and the ventricles are at rest (diastole). With atrial contraction, the final 30 percent of end-diastolic volume is provided. The preload is a major determinant of the amount of blood ejected during each ventricular contraction (stroke volume), that is, the greater the preload, the greater the stroke volume.

> This phenomenon illustrates Frank-Starling's Law: The more a striated muscle fiber is stretched, the more forcefully it will contract. A greater end-diastolic volume produces a greater stretching of myocardial fibers, which leads to a more forceful contraction, thus ejecting a greater stroke volume. This relationship continues only until a critical length is reached, following which, contraction is diminished. A graph of this concept is illustrated in Figure 6.3.

Figure 6.3   Graph Illustrating the Frank-Starling Law of the Heart
As we continue to increase the volume of blood in the ventricle at end-diastole (pre-load) the heart continues to eject approximately 50 percent of this amount because of the Frank-Starling Principle, that is, the greater the muscle is stretched, the more forcefully it contracts. This occurs only until the muscle's maximum capability to adapt is reached (point A). Continuing to increase diastolic filling beyond this point results in no further increase in stroke volume, and if continued, muscle contractility will begin to decrease (point B).

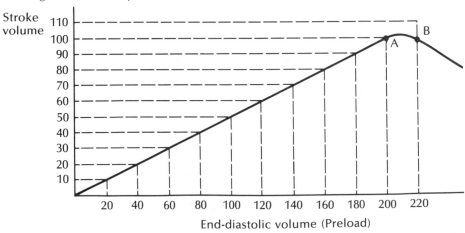

Events or drugs that alter the preload will obviously affect the stroke volume. Standing erect and motionless for prolonged periods will reduce venous return to the heart, thus decreasing stroke volume to the point that inadequate cerebral flow results in fainting.

After diastolic filling is completed, the contraction of the ventricles forces the blood against the AV valves closing them and producing the first heart sound (S_1), "lub." When this occurs, the only escape route for the blood is through the semilunar valves and out the aorta and the pulmonary artery. When the ventricles relax, blood in the aorta and the pulmonary artery backflows, thus closing the semilunar valves and creating the second heart sound (S_2), "Dup." Generally, 40 to 50 percent of the end-diastolic volume remains in the ventricle after systole and is appropriately termed the "end-systolic volume." Anything that impedes ventricular ejection of blood will increase myocardial wall tension and is referred to as being an "afterload factor." Such factors will decrease the stroke volume, thus increasing the blood volume left over, that is, end-systolic volume. Any factor that impedes flow through the aorta or the pulmonary arteries (afterload) may not only reduce stroke volume but also will definitely increase the work effort of the heart.

> Even in the healthy individual, moderate afterload increases may increase the end-systolic volume. However, this soon adds to the next end-diastolic volume, which further stretches the myocardium producing a more forceful contraction. In this manner, cardiac output does not suffer. However, this compensation may not be possible in diseased situations. As we will see in the next chapter, patients suffering heart failure and infarction are given drugs that reduce afterload as well as preload, thus reducing myocardial work effort. For this reason, it is of paramount importance that you understand these terms: preload, afterload, end-diastolic volume, and end-systolic volume (see Figures 6.4 and 6.5 on the next two pages).

BLOOD PRESSURE

Systolic blood pressure is primarily determined by cardiac output (rate × stroke volume) while diastolic pressure is determined by peripheral resistance. Since peripheral resistance is largely determined by the elasticity and the diameter of arterial vessels, dilating or constricting arteries has a major influence on diastolic pressure, while those drugs affecting the heart have a greater influence on cardiac output and, therefore, on systolic pressure. A common misconception is that a rapid pulse causes an increased pressure, when in fact, the opposite is actually

Figure 6.4.

A. During diastole, the ventricles fill with blood from the atria.

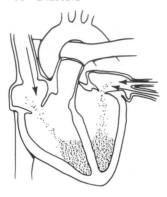

A   Diastole

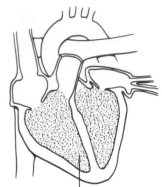

B   End of diastole

End-diastolic volume (preload)

B. At the end of this filling period, just as the ventricles begin to contract, the volume contained in the ventricles is referred to as the end-diastolic volume or "preload."

C. During ventricular systole, the amount of blood ejected through the aorta and the pulmonary artery is called the stroke volume.

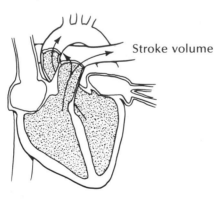

C   Systole

Stroke volume

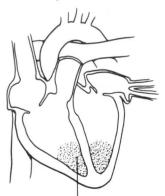

D   End of systole

End-systolic volume

D. The portion of the "preload" remaining in the ventricles after the stroke volume has been ejected is referred to as the end-systolic volume. Any factor that hinders the ejection of stroke volume and thus increases the amount of blood left in the ventricles (end-systolic volume) is referred to as an "afterload" factor.

more common. A slower pulse provides greater diastolic filling time, thus providing greater stroke volume and a sustained systolic pressure.

Rapid pulse rates are more commonly seen as a compensatory effort to generate a better cardiac output when the stroke volume is low, for example, in

---

Figure 6.5

A. Normal end-diastolic volume (EDV) is approximately 150 ml. Following ventricular systole, 75 ml of this is ejected as stroke volume (SV), and the remaining 75 ml is considered the end-systolic volume (ESV).

B. If increased "afterload" factors are introduced to impede ejection of stroke volume, a greater end-systolic volume results.

C. This increased ESV now adds to the next end-diastolic volume (175 ml). While the normal heart can adjust to this increased "preload" and eject a greater stroke volume (Starling's law), chronic afterload increase will eventually result in myocardial failure.

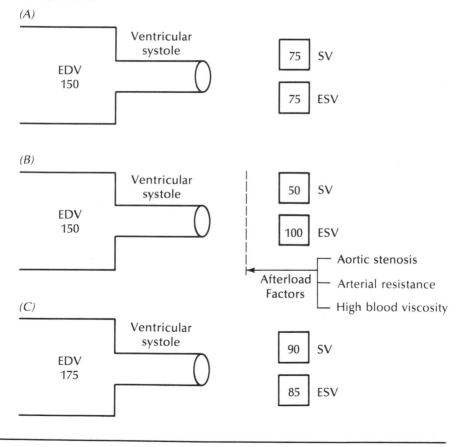

congestive failure. Rapid rates reduce diastolic filling and stroke volume, but may help maintain cardiac output and thus systolic pressure (see Figure 6.6).

Figure 6.6
Cardiac output is the amount of blood ejected by the heart each minute. This is calculated by multiplying the stroke volume times the heart rate.

A. If the amount of blood ejected by each ventricular contraction is 75 ml and this ejection occurs 72 times each minute, the cardiac output is 5.4 liters.

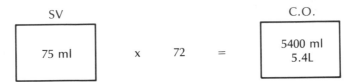

B. If a patient has a very strong heart, such as is the case with a well-conditioned athlete, the stroke volume is better and requires the heart to contract only 60 times a minute to produce the same cardiac output seen in A.

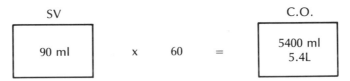

C. If the heart is not an efficient pump, such as is the case with a patient with congestive failure, the stroke volume is less, thereby requiring a rate of 90 to equal the 5.4 liters cardiac output. Since cardiac output is the major determinant of systolic blood pressure, you can see how both stroke volume and pulse cooperate in maintaining this pressure.

<table>
<tr><td>SV</td><td></td><td></td><td></td><td>C.O.</td></tr>
<tr><td>60 ml</td><td>x</td><td>90</td><td>=</td><td>5400 ml
5.4L</td></tr>
</table>

THE NEUROCONDUCTION SYSTEM

Well-designed laboratory studies illustrate the heart's automaticity witnessed by Edgar Allen Poe in the "Telltale Heart." While the autonomic nervous system alters heart rate and contractility, it can function independently of this innervation. Figure 6.7 illustrates the location of the four major components of this specialized system. Each portion can depolarize spontaneously, although the SA node enjoys dominance due to its greater rate.

The tissues of this system differ from typical neural tissue in two major ways. First of all, the membranes of these fibers are unable to maintain total impermeability to sodium and calcium ions. Whereas other neural cells must be stimulated to become permeable (see Chapter 2), the heart's neural tissues permit cations to slowly "leak" inwards until a spontaneous action potential occurs. This action potential is primarily caused by the influx of Ca^{++} in the SA and AV nodes but by Na^+ in the purkinjies. The second difference lies in the relationship to myocardial cells. In other neural tissue, the neural action potential is transmitted to the muscle cell by virtue of a neurotransmitter substance, that is, the neural fibers do not physically touch the muscle cell. In the heart, neuroconductive cells physically fuse with myocardial cells, allowing the action potential to spread directly from neural to contractile (muscle) cells.

Figure 6.7

The sinuatrial (SA) node depolarizes spontaneously 60 to 80 times each minute. This depolarization spreads along intra-atrial tracts to the atrioventricular (AV) node where the impulse is delayed briefly and then permitted to spread down the bundle of His node, through the Purkinjie fibers and onto the ventricular myocardial cells. The delay at the AV node is important since this allows time for the depolarization and the contraction of atrial muscle to occur before the impulse reaches the ventricles to stimulate their contraction.

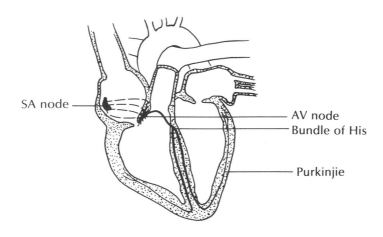

The sequence of electrical events is best understood when listed in the following manner:

1. The SA node depolarizes with its action potential spreading along intra-atrial tracts directly onto atrial muscle causing these cells to depolarize (see Figure 6.8A).
2. Following atrial muscle depolarization, these cells contract (atrial systole). While these events in the atrial muscle are occurring, the impulse originating at the SA node is spreading through the AV, down the bundles, through the purkinjies, and on to the ventricular myocardial cells resulting in their depolarization (see Figure 6.8B).
3. Following this depolarization, the ventricular myocardial cells contract (ventricular systole) (see Figure 6.8C).

Figure 6.8

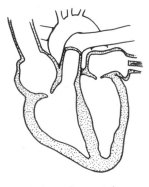 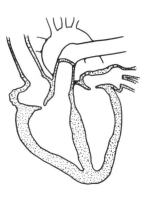 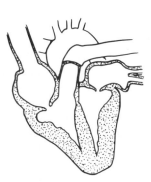

A. Atria and ventricles in diastole (relaxed)

B. Atria in systole but ventricles still in diastole

C. Atria in diastole but ventricles now in systole

The electrocardiogram (ECG) is used to analyze the events in the above sequence. The P-wave is produced by the depolarization of atrial muscle cells, while this same process in the ventricular myocardium is represented by the QRS complex. The T-wave represents the repolarization of the ventricular muscle. Notice that neither contraction or neuroconduction is represented by these waves. However, by analyzing Figure 6.9 you will see some of the deductions that we can make while visualizing an ECG recording. A patient's pulse is produced by contraction of the ventricles. If you palpate a patient's pulse while observing his or her ECG monitor, you will find the pulse to occur immediately *after* the peak of the QRS complex, not simultaneously. The waves of the ECG represent only depolarization and repolarization of muscle cells. Clinically, a patient can be in cardiac arrest and still produce a normal-looking ECG tracing!

The synopsis of cardiac function presented in this chapter must be fully understood if one is to grasp the concepts presented in the next chapter. Collectively, these drugs are able to modify every functional aspect of the cardiovascular system.

Figure 6.9

The P-wave represents atrial muscle depolarization. We may therefore assume that the SA node must have initiated the impulse prior to the P-wave (1) and the atrial muscle contracts immediately after atrial depolarization (2). The QRS complex represents depolarization of ventricular muscle. We may therefore assume that the ventricles contract immediately after they depolarize (4). If the SA node depolarizes at 1 and the ventricles begin to depolarize at 3, we then assume the interval between 1 and 3 to represent the spread of neural depolarization from the SA, through the AV, down the bundles, and into the purkinjies. This interval is commonly referred to as the "PR interval" and is prolonged if something delays the impulse from spreading through the AV node.

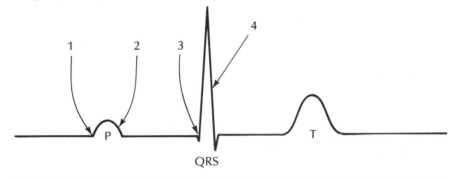

ARTICLES FOR DISCUSSION

1. **Littell, E. A.** 1981. Support responses of the cardiovascular system to exercise. *Physical Therapy* 61:1260–1264.
2. **Littell, E. A.** 1981. Neural regulation of cardiovascular response to exercise. *Physical Therapy* 61:1411–1418.
3. **Bollish, S. J., and Foster, T. S.** 1980. Swan-Ganz catheter: An important tool for monitoring drug therapy in the critically ill. *Hospital Formulary* 15:99.

7

Cardiovascular Pharmacology

A major reason for the increased life expectancy among United States residents is the advances in the treatment of cardiovascular disease. While public education and improved emergency medical service delivery have played vital roles, advances in pharmacotherapeutic agents must be considered paramount.

Like the autonomic nervous system, the cardiovascular system presents a challenging lesson in physiological principles. Having reviewed the salient features of this system, keep in mind that all drugs, including those discussed in this chapter, merely represent the attempt of scientists to interact with normal physiological processes.

HEART FAILURE

When the myocardium loses its inherent strength of contractility, it no longer functions as an effective pump. The consequences may be categorized as forward and backward failure. *Backward failure* represents the consequences of systemic and/or pulmonary venous congestion which occurs from inadequate flow of venous blood through the failing heart. *Forward failure* results from poor cardiac output leading to insufficient delivery of oxygenated blood to vital organs. In its most severe form, cardiogenic shock ensues.

Pharmacological management of heart failure consists of three primary goals:

1. Improving myocardial contractility.
2. Mobilizing edematous fluid.
3. Reducing myocardial workload.

Each of these goals may be accomplished by a specific group of cardiovascular agents.

75

Myocardial contractility is improved by digitalis glycoside preparations. Their cardiotonic effects include an increased force of contraction (positive inotropy), decreased rate (negative chronotropy), and decreased neuroconduction (negative dromotropy). The mechanism by which digitalis accomplishes these effects is quite complex, but it is significant that the positive inotropic mechanism is independent of beta-adrenergic receptors, that is, it is not reversed by propranolol.

> While numerous mechanisms are proposed for the inotropic mechanism, the most plausible is inhibition of the enzyme, sodium-potassium ATPase. This enzyme provides the energy for the sodium-potassium pump, which actively transports sodium extracellularly during the repolarization of myocardial membranes. As a result, Na^+ accumulates intracellularly, with myocardial cells possessing a unique mechanism for exchanging these excess sodium ions for extracellular calcium. By this complex series of events, digitalis is able to increase the levels of intracellular Ca^{++}, which are critical to the contractile mechanism.
>
> Negative chronotropic and dromotropic effects are diminished in heart preparations lacking parasympathetic innervation. This supports the hypothesis that these latter cardiotonic effects are produced, in part, by a central stimulation of vagal output.[1]

The failing myocardium obviously benefits from the positive inotropic effect, but one should also respect the benefit that occurs from the decrease in rate. This slower rate provides a greater diastolic filling period which, combined with the increase in contractility, can provide marked improvement in the stroke volume of a failing heart.

While digitalis rarely corrects atrial flutter or fibrillation, its negative dromotropic action on the AV node protects the ventricles from the rapid impulses generated in the atria. This capability renders digitalis preparations quite useful in the treatment of these atrial dysrhythmias.

Digitalis preparations produce several noncardiac side effects, the most notable being anorexia, nausea, and vomiting. However, their low therapeutic index is due to cardiac toxicity that generally stems from exaggerated chronotropic and dromotropic effects. Bradycardia and excessive AV nodal depression provide a great opportunity for ectopic pacemaker activity to develop, resulting in premature atrial and/or ventricular contractions (PVCs) and fibrillation. Digitalis toxicity is more likely to occur if serum potassium levels are low (hypokalemia), a condition often precipitated by diuretic agents. Because of the potential for cardiac toxicity, it is advisable to record the patient's pulse and, if applicable, observe his or her ECG monitor before administering any digitalis preparation.

Digoxin is the most widely employed cardiac glycoside. However, several preparations are available, differing mainly in their pharmacokinetic patterns (see Table 7.1).

TABLE 7.1 Digitalis preparations available in the United States

digitoxin	(Crystodigin, Purodigin)	deslanoside	(Cedilanid-D)
digoxin	(Lanoxin)	digitalis	(USP)
lanatoside C	(Cedilanid)	ouabain	(USP)

Another inotropic agent, dobutamine, is a unique catecholamine derivative that is gaining popularity in treating heart failure associated with acute myocardial infarction. It exerts its powerful inotropic effect by a beta-receptor mechanism and is unique among beta-adrenergics in that it produces minimal increases in heart rate.[2] While its rapid onset and brief duration of action offer certain advantages, the glycosides still remain the primary agents for increasing myocardial contractility.

A second goal in treating heart failure is to mobilize edematous fluids. This may be accomplished with agents that increase urination (diuresis). The subsequent reduction in both vascular and extravascular fluid volumes serves to reduce excessive workload on the failing pump. There are several classes of diuretic agents, each utilizing a unique mechanism to promote diuresis. However, the more commonly employed diuretics act by inhibiting the reabsorption of sodium in the renal tubules. The excretion of sodium thus creates an osmotic pressure favoring water excretion. Since hypokalemia is a common untoward effect of chronic diuretic use and serves to potentiate glycoside toxicity, it is not surprising that the most commonly prescribed diuretic for chronic use is a combination product containing a potassium-sparing diuretic along with a conventional thiazide derivative (Dyazide). Table 7.2 lists the more popular diuretic agents. Of these preparations, furosemide is the most efficacious and is the agent of choice in urgent situations. It is often referred to as a ''high-ceiling'' diuretic and, following intravenous administration, produces diuresis within 5 to 10 minutes.

Although diuretics provide some reduction in myocardial workload, acute situations frequently require the use of arterial and/or venous dilating drugs. Arterial dilation and subsequent afterload reduction is the primary effect of sodium nitroprusside (Nipride). While some venodilation occurs, it is generally agreed that nitroprusside is most active on arteriolar smooth muscle. Preload reduction is more readily accomplished by venous dilation using intravenous preparations of nitroglycerin. The nitrates are more commonly employed for episodes of angina pectoris and will be discussed more extensively later in this chapter.

TABLE 7.2   Commonly used diuretic preparations

A. *Osmotic agents* promote diuresis by acting as osmotically active solutes in the excreted urine.

   1. mannitol (Osmitrol)
   2. urea (Urevert)

B. *Natriuretic agents* promote excretion of sodium and chloride. The sodium excretion then attracts water osmotically. Most of these agents promote potassium excretion unless designated as "potassium-sparing."

   1. Thiazides
      a) chlorothiazide (Diuril)
      b) hydrochlorothiazide (Hydrodiuril)
      c) chlorthalidone (Hygroton)
   2. High-ceiling (very efficacious)
      a) furosemide (Lasix)
      b) ethacrynic acid (Edecrin)
   3. Potassium-sparing
      a) spironolactone (Aldactone)
      b) triamterene (Dyrenium)
   4. Combination Products
      a) triamterene and hydrochlorothiazide (Dyazide)
      b) spironolactone and hydrochlorothiazide (Aldactazide)

Table 7.3 below summarizes the pharmacological management of congestive heart failure.

TABLE 7.3   Summary of the pharmacotherapeutic management of heart failure

---

1. Improve force of contraction (contractility)
   a) digitalis glycosides
   b) dobutamine
2. Reduce edema and plasma volume, thus reducing work effort and venous congestion (preload and afterload)
   a) diuretic agents
3. Reduce afterload by reducing peripheral resistance (vasodilation)
   a) nitroprusside
   b) alpha blockers
   c) calcium channel blockers
4. Reduce preload by venous dilation
   a) nitroglycerin

ISCHEMIC HEART DISEASE

Inadequate coronary blood flow results in decreased nutrient and oxygen delivery to the myocardium. The major symptom of this disorder, *angina pectoris,* is often considered a disease, when actually this pain is merely a symptom of ischemia. The most common causes of myocardial ischemia are atherosclerosis and vaso-spasm of the coronary arteries. Should the blood flow deteriorate to a point where myocardial cells cannot survive, myocardial infarction occurs.

Since the drugs used for these disorders are often spoken of as "anti-anginal agents," one must keep in mind that they are not analgesics (painkillers), that is, the angina subsides only when ischemic conditions are improved. There are two logical ways to improve myocardial ischemia: improve coronary blood flow, and/ or decrease myocardial work effort so that blood supply is sufficient for myocardial needs.

The nitrate and nitrite preparations are the oldest and most popular drugs utilized in treating ischemic heart disease. They produce their beneficial effect primarily by causing venous dilation which decreases preload, that is, reduces myocardial work and, therefore, myocardial oxygen consumption. Although these agents are capable of producing coronary arterial dilation, this action is not considered clinically significant in most situations.

The mechanism by which nitrates induce smooth muscle relaxation is unknown. The reduction of preload by venous dilation is well-documented by numerous studies. Direct intracoronary injection fails to relieve angina symptoms, while reducing preload by phlebotomy does relieve these symptoms.[3] An exception occurs in those patients suffering from coronary artery spasm. In these patients, intravenous injection of nitroglycerin corrects the anginal episode by dilating coronary arteries.[4]

The prototype of the nitrates, nitroglycerin, is actually a misnomer. "Nitro" compounds contain direct carbon-to-nitrogen bonds, which accounts for their explosive character. The nitrates and the nitrites have oxygen atoms between the carbon and nitrogen atoms. Figure 7.1 compares the structure of the actual nitroglycerin molecule with that of glyceryl trinitrate, which is erroneously referred to as nitroglycerin.

The most common side effects seen in patients taking nitrate preparations are due to their vasodilating properties, that is, dizziness from mild hypotension and headache from vasodilation of cranial vessels. It is common for nitrates to be administered sublingually, but PO and topical routes are available. Table 7.4 lists the various available preparations.

Figure 7.1 Comparative structural formulas of nitroglycerin and glyceryl trinitrate.

```
        H                           H
        |                           |
   H — C — NO₂               H — C — O — NO₂
        |                           |
   H — C — NO₂               H — C — O — NO₂
        |                           |
   H — C — NO₂               H — C — O — NO₂
        |                           |
        H                           H
```

Nitroglycerin   Glyceryl trinitrate
                          (erroneously called nitroglycerin)

TABLE 7.4 Common nitrate preparations

glyceryl trinitrate	(Nitro-Bid, Nitrostat)
isosorbide dinitrate	(Isordil)
erythrityl tetranitrate	(Cardilate)

The *beta-blocking drugs* are also widely used for treating ischemic heart disease. By blocking the $beta_1$ cardiac receptor, the heart rate is decreased and thus work effort and myocardial oxygen requirements are reduced. Propranolol (Inderal) is the prototype of this group but produces some undesirable effects on other organs due to the $beta_2$ blockade. The most noteworthy of these side effects is bronchospasm in susceptible patients. For this reason, selective $beta_1$ blockers, such as metoprolol (Lopressor), are gaining popularity. Table 4.3 lists the presently employed beta-blocking agents.

It is critical to differentiate the mechanism by which the nitrates and the beta blockers reduce myocardial oxygen consumption. The former reduce preload via venous dilatation, while the beta blockers decrease heart rate. In those patients who suffer the coronary-spasm form of angina (Prinzmetal's angina), beta blockers may actually worsen the condition. By blocking beta receptors in coronary arteries, which mediate vasodilation, the alpha receptors present are unopposed and may result in more pronounced coronary vasospasm.[5]

The *calcium channel blockers* are an impressive group of cardiovascular agents whose indications are increasing at a staggering rate. The calcium ion has a major role in the contractile mechanism of all muscle cells, smooth, skeletal, and cardiac. Vascular smooth muscle relies on the steady inward "leak" of calcium since intracellular storage sites are quite limited. The name of this class of drugs delineates their mechanism, that is, they actually block the channels in smooth and cardiac muscle-cell membranes through which calcium must flow to enter the cytoplasm. In this manner the calcium channel blockers inhibit contraction, which results in relaxation or vasodilation. While these agents dilate most arterial systems, it is the coronary artery dilation that improves blood flow and proves particularly useful in vasospastic forms of angina.

> Although coronary dilation is considered the primary manner in which the calcium channel blockers improve ischemic symptoms, afterload reduction may also play a significant role. Relaxation of systemic arterial vessels lowers peripheral resistance, thus reducing the effort of the heart to eject blood from the ventricle.[6]

We will discuss additional uses of these agents later in this chapter. Presently, nifedipine (Procardia) is a popular member of this class used in treating vasospastic angina, with its most common side effect resulting from vasodilation-induced hypotension.

In summary, the major symptom of ischemic heart disease, angina pectoris, may be managed by drugs that either improve coronary blood flow or reduce myocardial work effort. Table 7.5 summarizes the pharmacological agents and their mechanisms. Notice that a reduction in myocardial work is the major beneficial effect of most agents.

TABLE 7.5 Summary of pharmacotherapeutic management of angina pectoris

---

A. Reduction of myocardial work by reducing venous return (preload)
   1. Nitrates and nitrites

B. Reduction of myocardial work by reducing heart rate
   1. Beta blockers

C. Reduction of myocardial work by systemic arterial dilation (afterload)
   1. Calcium channel blockers

D. Improving coronary blood flow by dilating coronary arteries
   1. Intravenous nitrates
   2. Calcium channel blockers

CARDIAC DYSRHYTHMIAS

Dysrhythmia is a general term used to describe any abnormal rate or rhythm in cardiac function. This term is preferred over "arrhythmia," which implies the absence of any rhythm, since this is not always the case. Cardiac dysrhythmias are caused by a variety of conditions ranging from stimulant ingestion to blockage along the neuroconductive pathway. While cardiac dysrhythmias represent an intriguing group of disorders, their exact nature and ECG interpretation are better explained elsewhere.[7, 8] For our purpose, let us understand that they all represent aberrant impulse formation and/or conduction within the heart's neuroconductive pathways and that they may result in diminished cardiac output.

Our goal in the pharmacological management of cardiac dysrhythmias is to reestablish normal electrical behavior (depolarization and repolarization) within the membranes of the neuroconductive cells. Each of the many antidysrhythmic drugs uses numerous complex mechanisms in generating their therapeutic effects. However, it has become quite common to categorize the many agents into four general classes based solely on their primary mechanism of action on cardiac neuroconductive tissues (see Table 7.6).

TABLE 7.6 Classification of antidysrhythmic agents and general indications for use

---

CLASS I

Mechanism:	Block inward flow of sodium ions ("local anesthetic"–type action).
Examples:	lidocaine (V)
	procainamide (S, V)
	quinidine (S, V)

CLASS II

Mechanism:	Block cardiac beta$_1$ receptor, thereby inhibiting sympathetic stimulation
Example:	propranolol (S, V)

CLASS III

Mechanism:	Prolong the duration of action potentials and therefore lengthen the effective refractory period
Example:	bretylium (V)

CLASS IV

Mechanism:	Block inward flow of calcium ions
Example:	verapamil (S)

S = supraventricular dysrhythmias   V = ventricular dysrhythmias

The Class I antidysrhythmics produce their effects primarily by blocking the inward flow of Na^+ during membrane depolarization. These sodium channel blockers actually employ a "local anesthetic"–type mechanism of action. Lidocaine, quinidine, and procainamide are the most popular members of this class.

As stated above, sodium channel blockade is only one of the mechanisms by which Class I agents produce their antidysrhythmic effect. In addition to sodium channel blockade, quinidine exerts a significant anticholinergic action, thus potentiating sympathetic stimulation to SA and AV nodal tissue. This action may prove counterproductive in suppressing atrial tachydysrhythmias. For this reason, digitalis is often administered prior to quinidine therapy. Since digitalis stimulates vagal innervation to the SA and AV node, quinidine's blocking action at these tissues will be less pronounced.[9]

The Class II agents produce their antidysrhythmic effects primarily by blocking the cardiac beta receptors. Beta blockers such as propranolol and metoprolol inhibit the stimulatory effect of the sympathetic nervous system, thereby attenuating any related dysrhythmic activity. Since beta-receptor availability is critical for myocardial contractility, cautious use of these agents is paramount when managing dysrhythmias in patients with concurrent heart failure.

The Class III antidysrhythmics are represented primarily by bretylium (Bretylol), an agent described as prolonging the duration of the action potential in purkinjie fibers. The significance of this mechanism is that as long as one action potential (impulse) is proceeding in a cell, the cell is refractory to another stimulus. In serious tachydysrhythmias, such as ventricular tachycardia and fibrillation, the purkinjies are being stimulated in rapid succession. Bretylium is able to prolong each action potential, thereby protecting the cells from continuous rapid stimuli.

Bretylium is structurally similar to sympathomimetic amines and produces a variety of hemodynamic effects. It initially triggers the release of norepinephrine from adrenergic terminals producing what is sometimes described as a "sympathetic storm." After approximately 20 minutes, bretylium reverses this action by actually inhibiting further norepinephrine release. Varying degrees of hypotension ensue, which accounts for the major side effect.[10]

The calcium channel blockers comprise the Class IV antidysrhythmic agents. Their vasodilator effects were discussed above along with their indication as antianginal agents. However, it must be remembered that calcium ions not only participate in smooth-muscle contraction but also participate in the action potential of neural tissues. This latter action is very significant in the depolarization phase of SA and AV nodal cells. For this reason, verapamil is very popular for treating supraventricular tachydysrhythmias, especially paroxysmal atrial tachycardia (PAT). The most notable side effects of the calcium channel blockers result from vasodilation, which results in varying degrees of hypotension. There is also some concern that their ability to block calcium entry to myocardial cells may decrease contractility in patients with heart failure.

> The calcium channel blockers represent one of the most promising advances in the treatment of cardiovascular disease. Since the inward flow of calcium ions is critical for the contraction of smooth and cardiac muscle as well as depolarization of SA and AV nodal tissue, the indications for these agents promise to increase over the next few years. Already their vasodilating capabilities are being expanded to include treatment of Raynaud's disease, hypertension, and cerebral vasospasm.[11, 12]

Some authorities advocate the adoption of two additional classes of antidysrhythmic agents to include the digitalis glycosides (Class V) and indirect cholinergic agents (Class VI). The ability of digitalis to slow SA and AV nodal conduction by its vagotonic action, makes it quite useful in protecting the ventricles from atrial flutter and fibrillation. Cholinesterase inhibitors such as edrophonium (Tensilon) produce a parasympathomimetic effect useful in slowing supraventricular tachycardias.

HYPERTENSION

Blood pressure is maintained by a combination of the factors illustrated in Figure 7.2. The pharmacological management of hypertension is designed to inhibit one or, more commonly, several of these factors.

Diuretic therapy is usually the initial selection (step 1) in most cases of hypertension. Its use in congestive heart failure was discussed previously, and the ability of diuretics to reduce plasma volume may partially explain their useful antihypertensive effect.

> The exact mechanism of their antihypertensive effect is not established. Although a reduction in plasma volume is a viable explanation for the initial reduction in pressure, the chronic effect cannot be explained by this mechanism. Sodium depletion seems to be the critical factor in sus-

taining a decreased peripheral resistance. The reduction in sodium levels may alter the alpha-receptor affinity of norepinephrine or may reduce the size of smooth-muscle cells in arterial walls, thus creating a wider vessel lumen.[13]

Figure 7.2 Blood pressure-controlling factors and sites of pharmacological interaction.

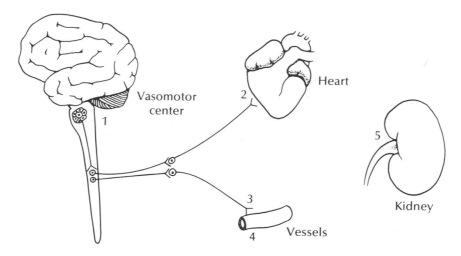

1. Depress vasomotor center—methyldopa.

2. Beta blockade—propranolol.

3. Inhibit neurotransmitter release—guanethidine.

4. Vasodilation—hydralazine.

5. Inhibit angiotensin II—captopril.

The inhibition of sympathetic outflow from the central nervous system will lower blood pressure. Indeed, mild elevation of pressure seen in anxiety states can be reduced somewhat by antianxiety medication (Valium, etc.). More specifically however, sympathetic outflow from the vasomotor center in the medulla is inhibited by an alpha-receptor subtype designated alpha.$_2$ Activation of this receptor by alpha$_2$ agonists decreases sympathetic outflow with a subsequent reduction in blood pressure. Methyldopa (Aldomet) and clonidine (Catapres) produce their antihypertensive effects by this mechanism. Since they exert their effects centrally, sedation is a common side effect produced by these preparations that is not seen with peripherally acting antihypertensive agents.

It would seem obvious that drugs capable of producing vasodilation will lower blood pressure and thus prove useful in treating hypertension. On this basis, many vasodilators are used in contemporary antihypertensive therapy. The mechanisms by which vasodilation is produced may be conveniently divided into three categories:

1. Direct relaxation of vascular smooth muscle is the mechanism by which hydralazine (Apresoline) produces its antihypertensive effect. The precise intracellular mechanism resulting in the relaxation has not been established.
2. Blockade of alpha receptors on arterial and venous walls prevents norepinephrine access to exert its vasoconstrictive action. Prazosin (Minipress) is a popular agent utilizing this principle.
3. Drugs are available which prevent the uptake and/or the release of norepinephrine from peripheral and central adrenergic nerve endings. By these mechanisms, reserpine (Serpasil) and guanethidine (Ismelin) prevent sympathetic-induced vasoconstriction.

The beta-blocking agents are quite popular as antihypertensive agents. Certainly, their ability to reduce cardiac output by blocking sympathetic cardiac stimulation accounts for a portion of their antihypertensive effect. However, undefined CNS mechanisms are also considered likely.

The renin-angiotensin system plays a vital role in blood pressure regulation. Renin is an enzyme released from the juxtaglomerular cells in the kidney and functions to catalyze the initial step in the formation of angiotensin II (see Figure 7.3). Renin release is triggered by low blood pressure, hyponatremia, and sympathetic innervation (beta$_2$ receptor). Angiotensin II elevates blood pressure in two

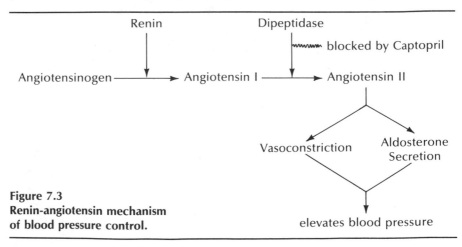

Figure 7.3
**Renin-angiotensin mechanism
of blood pressure control.**

manners, direct vasoconstriction and stimulation of aldosterone secretion. Conversion of angiotensin I to angiotensin II can be prevented by inhibiting the converting enzyme, peptidyl dipeptidase (PDP). It follows that the PDP inhibitor, captopril (Capoten), produces its antihypertensive effect in this manner.

> It is important that one recognize that captopril does not directly inhibit the release of renin from the kidney. Its mechanism is exerted later in the angiotensin synthetic pathway. However, there is great interest in the possibility that the inhibition of renin release may account for additional anithypertensive mechanisms produced by clonidine and beta-adrenergic blocking agents.[14, 15]

Many hypertensive patients are managed by concurrent therapy with two or three of the antihypertensive agents described above. The selections differ in their mechanism of action and therefore provide an excellent example of useful synergistic actions. Typically a patient with *mild* hypertension is treated with a diuretic and/or a beta blocker. If this regimen proves ineffective, or if the patient suffers *moderate* hypertension, one of the vasodilators is added. Vasodilator therapy commonly requires concurrent beta blocker use to prevent the reflex tachycardia that is likely to follow vasodilation. The centrally acting agents and guanethidine are generally utilized in more refractory cases. Regardless of their mechanism, all medications designed to lower blood pressure may produce postural hypotension as a common side effect. Figure 7.2 summarizes the antihypertensive mechanisms of the popular preparations.

ANTICOAGULANTS

The ultimate product in the coagulation pathway is fibrin. The complex reactions between factors in the cascade preceding fibrin formation are actually a series of enzymes, each serving to catalyze the formation of the next enzyme in the cascade. One series of enzymes is found in the circulating blood and is referred to as the intrinsic system or pathway. The second series is found in the tissues and is appropriately termed the extrinsic system. Figure 7.4 illustrates that both extrinsic and intrinsic cascades meet to convert the Stuart factor (Factor X) to its activated enzymatic form, Factor Xa. From this point, through fibrin formation, the cascade is a common pathway. For adequate amounts of activated Stuart factor (Xa) to be formed, both extrinsic and intrinsic pathways must be functional. Inhibiting critical steps in this pathway is the manner in which anticoagulant drugs prevent fibrin formation.

Anticoagulants are employed for the prevention of thromboembolic disorders. The word "prevention" must be emphasized. These drugs lack thrombolytic capability and must be used prophylactically in those situations where patients are predisposed to thromboembolus formation, for example, surgery, deep venous phlebitis, and rheumatic heart disease.

Heparin is naturally present in human mast cells, but its physiological significance is unknown. Commercial preparations have 10 to 20 times the anticoagulant activity of this natural form. Heparin produces its anticoagulant effect indirectly by potentiating the inhibitory action of antithrombin III on several activated clotting factors, most significantly Xa and thrombin (see Figure 7.4).

Intermittent intravenous administration and subcutaneous injections represent the common methods of administering heparin to hospitalized patients. Its inhibitory activity may be reversed by protamine should hemorrhage occur.

The oral anticoagulants were discovered quite accidentally when a chemical found in spoiled clover produced a hemorrhagic disorder in cattle. The chemical was identified as bishydroxycoumarin and, following its successful use as a rodenticide, was found to be therapeutically useful in human clotting disorders. While several derivatives are available, warfarin is the major generic compound utilized and is available under the brand names Coumadin and Panwarfin.

Figure 7.4 Final portions of coagulation cascade.
Circled factors are dependent on vitamin K for synthesis and are thus inhibited by warfarin preparations.

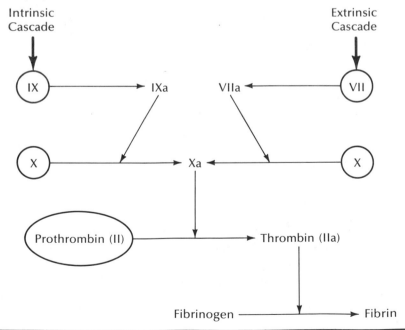

> *Warfarin* presents an interesting example of how generic and brand names are selected. It is an acronym for the developing company, *Wisconsin Alumni Research Foundation*. To these initials they added the suffix of the parent compound, bishydroxycoum*arin* to produce Warfarin.

Warfarin is a vitamin K antagonist and thus prevents the formation of those factors dependent on vitamin K for synthesis (see Figure 7.4). As you might suppose, administering vitamin K to a "warfarinized" patient will counteract the anticoagulant effect. However, even following intravenous administration of phytonadione (vitamin K_1), it takes the liver several hours to synthesize the new factors.

Hemorrhage is the most profound adverse effect of all anticoagulant preparations. Patients maintained on chronic warfarin therapy must have prothrombin times analyzed on a regular basis to assure proper warfarin levels. Caution must be exercised when handling these patients since even minor trauma may result in severe hemorrhage. Of equal significance is the multitude of drugs that antagonize and potentiate the anticoagulant effect of warfarin and heparin preparations. While too numerous to expound upon, one should check the potential of adverse interactions prior to administering any medication to a patient on anticoagulant therapy. Worth mention are the aspirinlike drugs because of their widespread use. These drugs prevent platelet aggregation which, combined with the anticoagulant's inhibition of fibrin formation, prolongs bleeding time dramatically. Additionally, these drugs erode mucous membranes, which promotes hemorrhage. Acetaminophen (Tylenol, others) is the substitute of choice for patients receiving anticoagulant therapy.

SUMMARY

Even an introductory synopsis such as this presents a formidable challenge for any student. A second, and perhaps a third, reading will be necessary to grasp the pertinent concepts of cardiovascular pharmacology. By understanding these concepts you will have a better grasp of the patient's medical condition as well as the pharmacological goals and hazards of therapy.

SYNOPSIS OF THERAPEUTIC AGENTS

I. Cardiac glycosides

A. ACTION
1. Increase force
2. Decrease rate
3. Decrease AV conduction

B. COMMON INDICATIONS
1. Congestive heart failure
2. Atrial flutter, fibrillation

C. PREPARATIONS
1. Digoxin (Lanoxin)

D. SECONDARY EFFECTS
1. Noncardiac
   a) Nausea
   b) Anorexia
2. Cardiac
   a) Bradycardia
   b) AV block
   c) Atrial and/or ventricular ectopy
   d) Virtually any dysrhythmia

II. Nitrates

A. ACTION
1. Venous dilation results in reduced preload and therefore reduced workload

B. COMMON INDICATIONS
1. Angina pectoris
2. Congestive heart failure

C. PREPARATIONS
1. Glyceryl trinitrate (nitroglycerin)

D. SECONDARY EFFECTS
1. Headache
2. Dizziness (from hypotension)

III. Antidysrhythmics

A. ACTION
   1. Depress excitatory impulses within cardiac neuroconductive pathway
B. COMMON INDICATIONS
   1. Various cardiac dysrhythmias
C. PREPARATIONS
   1. Local anesthetics (lidocaine)
   2. Beta blockers (propranolol)
   3. Calcium blockers (verapamil)
D. SECONDARY EFFECTS
   1. Excessive cardiac depression

IV. Diuretics

A. ACTION
   1. Diuresis
B. COMMON INDICATIONS
   1. Edema from any cause (CHF, etc.)
   2. Hypertension
C. PREPARATIONS
   1. Chlorothiazide (Diuril)
D. SECONDARY EFFECTS
   1. Hypokalemia
   2. Dehydration

V. Vasodilators

A. ACTION
   1. Produce arterial dilation by a variety of local and central mechanisms
B. COMMON INDICATIONS
   1. Hypertension
   2. Congestive heart failure

SYNOPSIS OF THERAPEUTIC AGENTS *(continued)*

V. Vasodilators *(continued)*

    C. PREPARATIONS

        1. Hydralazine (Apresoline)

        2. Prazosin (Minipress)

        3. Alpha methyldopa (Aldomet)

    D. SECONDARY EFFECTS

        1. Postural hypotension

VI. Beta blockers

    A. ACTION

        1. Decrease sympathetic stimulation to the heart

    B. COMMON INDICATIONS

        1. Angina

        2. Hypertension

        3. Dysrhythmias

    C. PREPARATIONS

        1. Propranolol (Inderal)

    D. SECONDARY EFFECT

        1. Bronchospasm

VII. Calcium channel blockers

    A. ACTION

        1. Inhibit calcium entry to neural, smooth, and cardiac muscle cells

    B. COMMON INDICATIONS

        1. Atrial dysrhythmias

        2. Angina

    C. PREPARATIONS

        1. Verapamil (Isoptin)

    D. SECONDARY EFFECTS

        1. Hypotension

VIII. Anticoagulants

    A. ACTION
        1. Inhibit coagulation pathway
    B. COMMON INDICATIONS
        1. Thromboembolic disorders
    C. PREPARATIONS
        1. Heparin
        2. Warfarin (Coumadin)
    D. SECONDARY EFFECTS
        1. Hemorrhage

ARTICLES FOR DISCUSSION

1. **Rasmussen, S. R., et al.** 1975. The pharmacology and clinical use of digitalis. *Cardiovascular Nursing* 11:23–28.
2. **Albeit, S., et al.** 1977. Recognizing digitalis toxicity. *American Journal of Nursing* 77:1935–1945.
3. **Reeder, J. M.** 1982. Understanding Von Willebrand's disease. *AORN Journal* 35:1310–1319.
4. **Lapinski, M. L.** 1982. Cardiovascular drugs and the elderly population. *Heart and Lung* 11:430–434.
5. **Kessler, K. M.** 1980. Pharmacological basis of cardiovascular drug action. *Hospital Formulary* 15:457.
6. **Ram, C. V.** 1981. Diuretics in the treatment of hypertension. *Hospital Formulary* 16:741.
7. **Finnerty, F. A.** 1979. Step 2 regimens in hypertension: Assessment. *JAMA* 241:579.
8. **Ross, L. P., and Antman, E. M.** 1983. Calcium channel blockers: New treatment for cardiovascular disease. *American Journal of Nursing* 83:382–387.
9. **Gaskins, J. D., et al. 1982.** Comparative review of intravenous nitroglycerin and nitroprusside sodium. *Hospital Formulary* 17:928–934.
10. **Drayer, J. I., and Weber, M. A.** 1983. Current concepts in the evaluation and treatment of patients with mild to moderate hypertension. *Hospital Formulary* 18:164–170.

11. **Purcell, J. A. and Holder, C. K.** 1982. Intravenous nitroglycerin. *American Journal of Nursing* 82:254–259.

12. **Abrams, J.** 1980. Nitroglycerin and long-acting nitrates. *New England Journal of Medicine* 302:1234.

13. **Johnson, G. P., and Johanson, B. C.** 1983. Beta blockers: An expert's guide to what's on the market. *American Journal of Nursing* 83:1034–1043.

14. **Braker, D. C.** 1984. Clinical utility of the potassium-sparing diuretics. *Hospital Formulary* 19:79–82.

REFERENCES

1. **Mason, D. T.** 1974. Digitalis pharmacology and therapeutics: Recent advances. *Annals of Internal Medicine* 80:520–530.

2. **Goldstein, R. A., et al.** 1980. A comparison of digoxin and dobutamine in patients with acute infarction and cardiac failure. *New England Journal of Medicine* 303:846–849.

3. **Parker, J. D., et al.** 1970. The influence of changes in blood volume on angina pectoris: A study of effect of phlebotomy. *Circulation* 16:593–604.

4. **Straver, B. E., and Scherpe, A.** 1978. Ventricular functions and coronary hemodynamics after intravenous nitroglycerin in coronary artery disease. *American Heart Journal* (St. Louis) 95:210–219.

5. **Hillis, L. D., and Braunwald, E.** 1978. Coronary artery spasm. *New England Journal of Medicine* 13:695–702.

6. **Stone, P. H., et al.** 1980. Calcium channel blocking agents in the treatment of cardiovascular disorders. Part II: Hemodynamic effects and clinical applications. *Annals of Internal Medicine* 93:886–904.

7. **Dubin, D.** 1978. *Rapid Interpretation of EKGs,* 3rd ed., Tampa: Cover Publishing Co.

8. **Phillips, R. E., and Feeney, M. K.** 1973. *The Cardiac Rhythms*. Philadelphia: W. B. Saunders.

9. **Goodman, L. S., and Gilman, A.** 1980. *The Pharmacological Basis of Therapeutics*. 6th ed. New York: Macmillan, p. 773.

10. **Koch-Weser, J.** 1979. Drug therapy: Bretylium. *New England Journal of Medicine* 300:473–477.

11. **Reves, J. G., et al.** 1982. Calcium entry blockers: Uses and implications for anesthesiologists. *Anesthesiology* 57:504–518.

12. **Rodeheffer, R. J., et al.** 1983. Controlled double-blind trial of Nifedipine in the treatment of Raynaud's phenomenon. *New England Journal of Medicine* 308:880–883.

13. Tobian, L. 1967. Why do thiazide diuretics lower blood pressure in essential hypertension? *Annual Review of Pharmacology* (Palo Alto) 7:399–408.

14. Bowman, W. C., and Rand, M. J. 1980. *Textbook of Pharmacology,* 2nd ed. pg 23.40, St. Louis: Blackwell Mosby Book Distributors.

15. Weber, M. A., et al. 1978. The effects of clonidine and propranolol, separately and in combination, on blood pressure and plasma renin activity in essential hypertension. *Journal of Clinical Pharmacology* 18:233–234.

8

The Central Nervous System

Microscopically, the central nervous system (CNS) resembles the peripheral nervous system (PNS) in that it is comprised of the same structural and functional units—neurons. While these neurons have a variety of shapes and complex interrelationships, they are still grouped together forming structures analogous to the ganglia and the nerves of the peripheral nervous system. The nomenclature differs in that the clusters of cell bodies are termed nuclei instead of ganglia and the bundles of axons are called tracts instead of nerves. Like the peripheral nervous system, the performance of this central system of neurons is predicated on the release of a variety of neurotransmitters that will be discussed throughout this chapter.

The CNS may be separated into three distinct portions: higher brain, lower brain, and spinal cord (see Figure 8.1).

TABLE 8.1   Brain regions and general functions

Higher Brain

Cerebral cortex	Processes all incoming impulses, stores them (memory), and supervises the function of most other brain regions.

Lower Brain

Basal ganglia and extrapyramidal system	Depresses involuntary movements in concert with pyramidal tracts from the cortex.
Thalamus	Regulates and relays information to the cortex and other regions. May be viewed as the cortex's "principal vice-president."
Hypothalamus	Controls autonomic nervous system, adenohypophyseal hormones, body temperature, and emotions.
Medulla oblongata	Controls respiratory and vasomotor functions, vomiting reflex, and cortical arousal levels (RAS).
Cerebellum	Maintains or stabilizes body posture.

Figure 8.1 General divisions of the central nervous system.
Only the cortex of the cerebrum comprises the higher brain.

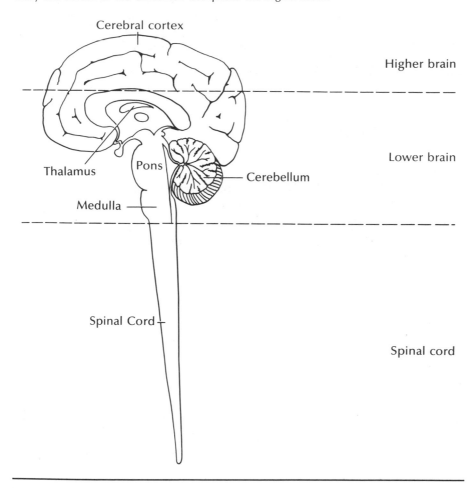

The higher brain consists of the cerebral cortex. This portion may be likened to a computer which not only stores and remembers our many experiences but influences and interprets the many independent functions of the lower brain and the spinal cord.

The lower brain consists of many tracts and nuclei comprising the remainder of the cerebrum, as well as the thalamus, hypothalamus, medulla, pons, and cerebellum. Their functions may be collectively categorized as "subconscious functions" and are listed in Table 8.1.

The spinal cord is actually an "extension cord" which neurally connects the brain with the remainder of our body. While it is able to perform many reflex functions independently from the brain, it primarily receives impulses from, or sends impulses to, the various brain centers.

The goal of this chapter is to provide a basis for understanding those drugs which alter CNS function. At this point it would be wise to take a closer look at the specific brain regions that serve as target sites for primary and/or secondary drug actions. You may refer to Figure 8.1 for an appreciation of the gross anatomical location of each of these areas.

MEDULLA

The respiratory center lies within the medulla oblongata and is comprised of several sets of neurons which control inspiration, expiration, and respiratory rate. A very important group of chemosensitive neurons regulate the activity of these former neurons. They are very sensitive to blood CO_2 levels (pCO_2) and function to stimulate inspiratory neurons when CO_2 levels are high. Sedative and narcotic drugs may depress these chemosensitive neurons, leading to varying degrees of respiratory depression.

> Actually these neurons are sensitive to hydrogen ion concentrations, not the CO_2 molecule. However, since the blood-brain barrier is relatively impermeable to hydrogen ions, we generally consider CO_2 levels as the stimulus for respiratory drive. Carbon dioxide readily diffuses across the blood-brain barrier and reacts with water to form carbonic acid, which in turn supplies the hydrogen ions to stimulate the chemosensitive neurons.
>
> $$CO_2 + H_2O \longrightarrow H_2CO_3 \longrightarrow H^+ + HCO_3^-$$

Also located in the medulla is a system of neurons referred to as the vasomotor control center. These neurons control heart rate and blood vessel diameter, and therefore have significant control over blood pressure. Although this area is under the control of higher brain centers, such as the hypothalamus and the cortex, pharmacological agents which depress medullary function may produce serious cardiovascular depression.

The chemoreceptor trigger zone is comprised of a group of neurons which release primarily dopamine as a neurotransmitter. When activated, these neurons stimulate the vomiting center to discharge impulses along the glossopharyngeal and vagal pathways, which stimulate emetic activity in the gastrointestinal tract. This vomiting center may also be activated by afferent neurons traveling with various cranial nerves (see Figure 8.2).

Figure 8.2

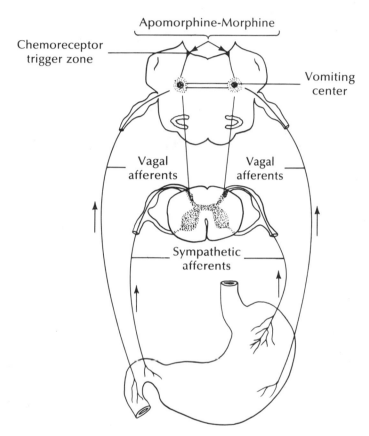

The chemoreceptor trigger zone and vomiting center are located in the medulla oblongata. (From Guyton, A.C., 1981. *Textbook of Medical Physiology*. Philadelphia: W. B. Saunders.)

The action of many of the drugs known to produce nausea results from their stimulation of this chemotrigger zone. Conversely, the efficacy of many popular antiemetic (antinausea) drugs is based on their ability to block dopamine receptors in this region.

RETICULAR ACTIVATING SYSTEM

The reticular activating system (RAS) is a group of neuronal tracts that extend from the brain stem (pons and medulla) through the thalamus and branches into most areas of the cerebral cortex. It must not be viewed as a distinct anatomical portion such as the medulla or the hypothalamus. Instead it is recognized and named according to the function it performs, activating the cerebral cortex. It is this system of neurons that determines the degree of "wakefulness" or "alertness" of the cortical areas.

It is generally accepted that sedative drugs such as barbiturates, produce their primary effect by depressing the neurons of the reticular activating system. By this action, the cortical functions become depressed due to lack of stimulation from the RAS.

BASAL GANGLIA

By strict definition the basal ganglia should be referred to as the "basal nuclei" since they represent a group of neural cell bodies lying within the central nervous system. However, the former terminology is so well-established that a change is unlikely.

Anatomically, the basal ganglia are a collection of nuclei scattered throughout portions of the brain stem, hypothalamus, thalamus, and cerebrum. The processes of these cell bodies form numerous tracts within the brain and the spinal cord which are collectivelly referred to as the extrapyramidal tracts.

The physiological activity of this system is very complex and poorly understood. However, its overall inhibitory role on skeletal muscle activity is well-accepted and serves to regulate discordant, involuntary skeletal muscle movement. The biochemical basis for this function rests on a delicate balance between the neurotransmitters, acetylcholine (excitatory) and dopamine (inhibitory). It seems that excitatory neurons which release acetylcholine are inhibited by neurons which release dopamine.

Parkinson's disease, or paralysis agitans, is a dopamine-deficiency state in which the patient exhibits varying degrees of tremor, muscle rigidity, and other uncontrolled skeletal muscle activity. These symptoms result from the fact that the excitatory neurons releasing acetylcholine are not being inhibited by the dopaminergic neurons. The condition may be pharmacologically improved by replacing dopamine stores with the synthetic precursor, L-dopa, and/or blocking the excitatory cholinergic effects with centrally acting anticholinergic drugs.

Parkinsonian symptoms may be produced as a secondary effect by a variety of antipsychotic drugs by virtue of their dopamine-receptor–blocking capability. In essence, these drugs produce a temporary "dopamine deficiency state."

LIMBIC SYSTEM

The limbic system consists of many tracts and nuclei scattered throughout the subcortical region of the cerebrum and the lower brain. At the center of this system is the hypothalamus, which is considered to be the primary motor output of this system. Vegetative functions (thirst, hunger, etc.) and emotional behavior are the major products of this system.

Psychiatric disorders are related to the dysfunction of this system and seem to correlate with abnormal levels of the neurotransmitters norepinephrine, serotonin, dopamine, and acetylcholine. Agents that increase norepinephrine and serotonin levels, such as tricyclic antidepressants, seem to elevate mood; and those blocking dopamine receptors, such as major tranquilizers, depress manic episodes.

PAIN PATHWAYS

Following their stimulation, pain receptors trigger an impulse which travels through pain fibers of spinal nerves to the spinal cord. In the cord, the fibers synapse with the cell bodies of internuncial neurons located in an area called the substantia gelatinosa. Axons originating in this area form ascending tracts, that is, spinothalamic tracts, which travel to the thalamus where additional synapses send the impulse to the cerebral cortex, hypothalamus, and other areas of the brain (see Figure 8.3 overleaf).

Scattered throughout the pathway described above are neurons whose neurotransmitters depress pain-impulse transmission and/or impulse interpretation. These neurotransmitters resemble morphine in action and are referred to as *endorphins* and *enkephalins*. The analgesic effect of narcotic agents is produced by their interaction with receptors at these locations.

SUMMARY

This review must not be viewed as a precise presentation of central nervous system structure and function. Instead, it was designed to provide the fundamental groundwork for understanding centrally acting drugs. Many of the concepts presented will be expanded as we discuss the specific drug groups that follow. Since all of these drugs interact with CNS neurotransmitters and/or their receptors, Table 8.2 offers a brief synopsis of CNS neurotransmitter location and function.

Figure 8.3 **The pain pathway from the spinal cord to the cerebral cortex.**

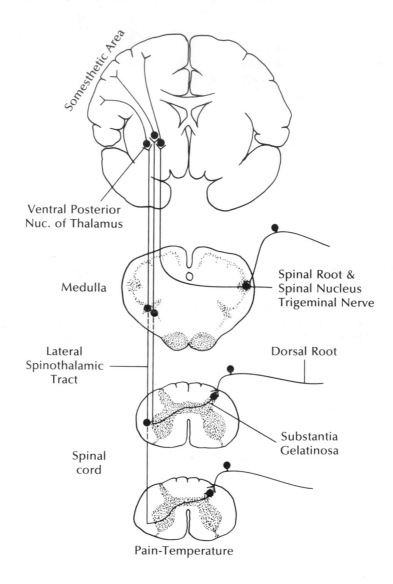

Illustration from Clark, R.G., 1970. *Manter and Gatz's Clinical Neuroanatomy and Neurophysiology,* 5th ed., Philadelphia: F. A. Davis.

TABLE 8.2   CNS neurotransmitters and proposed functions

Neurotransmitter	Proposed Function
Gamma-aminobutyric acid	Produces sedation and other inhibitory actions
Glycine	Decreases anxiety and skeletal muscle tone
Acetylcholine	Triggers extrapyramidal movements and generalized CNS arousal
Dopamine	Triggers vomiting reflex and manic behavior and inhibits extrapyramidal movements
Norepinephrine	Decreases appetite and facilitates memory, learning, and attention
5-Hydroxytryptamine (serotonin)	Alters behavior
Endorphins and enkephalins	Increases pain tolerance
Epinephrine, histamine, others	Unknown

9

Sedative-Hypnotics and Anticonvulsants

Terminology used to classify this class of drugs is not so unique as pharmaceutical companies would lead you to believe. Antianxiety (calming), sedation (drowsiness), and hypnosis (a state of sleep) are descriptive terms related more to dosage than to unique pharmacological mechanisms. Indeed a drug, such as phenobarbital, may produce a calming effect at low dosages and drowsiness at greater dosages and facilitate the onset of sleep at higher-dose ranges (see Figure 9.1).

Figure 9.1   Dose-response curve exemplary of most sedative-hypnotic preparations.

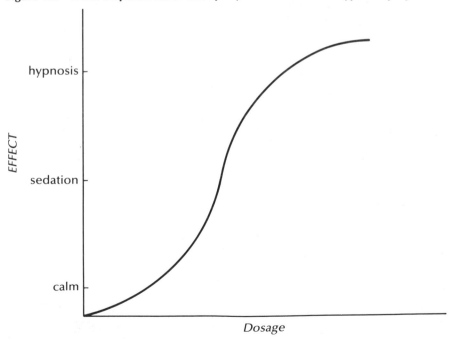

Sedative-hypnotics produce similar primary and secondary effects differing primarily in the frequency and the intensity of each effect (see Table 9.1).

TABLE 9.1   Effects and indications for most sedative-hypnotic preparations

Useful Primary Effects	Undesirable Effects	Indications
anxiolytic	depress REM sleep	anxiety
sedation	dependence	insomnia
hypnosis	paradoxical CNA stimulation	seizures
anticonvulsant (barbiturates, benzodiazepines)	respiratory and cardiovascular depression	muscle spasm
skeletal muscle relaxation (benzodiazepines)		

BARBITURATES

The barbiturates were the first chemical group in which numerous compounds were synthesized for therapeutic use. Their exact mechanism of action is not well-established, but some evidence exists for a GABA-like mechanism similar to the benzodiazepine preparations (see below).[1]

As a group, the barbiturates should be viewed as possessing the lowest therapeutic index and thus, are the most likely to produce the undesired effects listed in Table 9.1. While several methods exist for classifying the members of this group, Table 9.2 lists popular preparations according to their duration of effect and indications for use.

TABLE 9.2   Barbiturate preparations listed according to duration of effect and popular indications

Classification	Duration	Example	Indication
ultrashort	5–10 minutes	thiopental (Pentothal)	general anesthesia
short	4–6 hours	pentobarbital (Nembutal) secobarbital (Seconal)	insomnia, preoperative
intermediate	6–12 hours	amobarbital (Amytal)	insomnia, seizures
long	12–24 hours	phenobarbital (Luminal)	anxiety, seizures

BENZODIAZEPINES

This chemical group presently enjoys the greatest popularity of the sedative-type drugs. This status is well-deserved since their efficacy and safety is unsurpassed by other groups. (Of course the intense marketing strategies employed by pharmaceutical companies are equally notable.)

It is somewhat ironic that the youngest of all sedative groups should be so well-understood in terms of the mechanism of action. All members of this group are thought to produce their sedative effect by potentiating the depressant action of the inhibitory neurotransmitter, gamma-aminobutyric acid (GABA).[2]

There is considerable evidence to support distinct mechanisms for the sedative, anticonvulsant, antianxiety, and skeletal-muscle relaxant properties of the benzodiazepines.

Benzodiazepine receptors have been identified in close approximation to GABA receptors. When a benzodiazepine binds to its receptor, the GABA receptor becomes more receptive to its neurotransmitter, gamma-aminobutyric acid. This latter action produces anticonvulsant and sedative effects. Realize that if the patient were to be "GABA-less," benzodiazepines would be without effect.

There is also evidence that benzodiazepines bind to glycine receptors in the brainstem, where the antianxiety and skeletal muscle-relaxant effects are putatively produced.[2]

Diazepam (Valium) may be considered the prototype benzodiazepine and has enjoyed the distinction of being among the five most frequently prescribed drugs for many years. Most often it is used for its muscle-relaxant and antianxiety effects but also preoperatively for a wide range of medical and dental procedures. In striking contrast to the barbiturates, the benzodiazepines may be considered least likely to produce the undesired effects shared by the sedative-type drugs. The various benzodiazepines differ in the rate of onset and the duration of action but are all quite comparable in sedative and anxiolytic (antianxiety) efficacy. A major pharmacokinetic difference among preparations is the presence or absence of active metabolites which may permit cumulative effects following chronic use. Table 9.3 lists the popular benzodiazepine preparations.

ANTIHISTAMINES

This group of drugs will be discussed more extensively in Chapter 15 where sedation will be mentioned as their major secondary effect. However, hydroxyzine

TABLE 9.3   Benzodiazepine preparations comparing typical clinical uses and presence of active metabolites*

Preparations	Significant active metabolites	Anxiety	Insomnia	Seizure disorders
alprazolam (Xanax)	0	+	0	0
chlordiazepoxide (Librium)	+	+	0	0
clonazepam (Clonopin)	0	0	0	+
clorazepate (Tranxene)	+	+	0	+
diazepam (Valium)	+	+	0	+
flurazepam (Dalmane)	+	0	+	0
halazepam (Paxipam)	+	+	0	0
lorazepam (Ativan)	0	+	+	0
oxazepam (Serax)	0	+	0	0
prazepam (Centrax)	+	+	0	0
temazepam (Restoril)	0	0	+	0
triazolam (Halcion)	0	0	+	0

*(adapted from *AMA Drug Evaluations,* 5th ed., 1983)

(Vistaril) is one antihistamine whose clinical use is almost exclusively based on its sedative properties. It has a high therapeutic index and is quite popular in pre-operative medication regimens, especially in combination with narcotics such as meperidine (Demerol). Additionally, hydroxyzine is widely used by pediatric physicians and dentists (pedodontists) to calm anxious children during treatment. The mechanism by which these agents produce their sedative effect is poorly defined, but may be related to their efficacy as central histamine antagonists. This concept will be addressed further in Chapter 15.

MISCELLANEOUS AGENTS

There are many sedative agents that defy convenient classification and must be mentioned under this collective heading. (Certainly the benzodiazepines, antihistamines, and barbiturates offer more than adequate numbers of preparations to treat our nation's anxiety and insomnia, but the marketing principle of "supply versus demand" allows a place for numerous miscellaneous agents.) At one time, the agents listed in Table 9.4 were considered quite essential but have declined in popularity with the introduction of so many benzodiazepine preparations.

TABLE 9.4 Antihistamines and other miscellaneous sedative agents

chloral hydrate (Noctec)	hydroxyzine (Atarax, Vistaril)
ethchlorvynol (Pacidyl)	meprobamate (Equanil, Miltown)
ethinamate (Valmid)	methaqualone (Quaalude)
glutethimide (Doriden)	promethazine (Phenergan)

ANTICONVULSANT DRUGS

Many sedative preparations possess varying degrees of anticonvulsant activity. The more efficacious agents are used exclusively for this effect and, while conveniently classified as anticonvulsants, their sedative properties account for their most prevalent side effect.

> Terminology is this area is often used erroneously. A "seizure" implies a sudden but transient episode of abnormal neurological activity. All types of neural tissue may participate, but when motor neurons are hyperactive, the seizure is described as being "convulsive." If seizure episodes occur on a chronic basis, the term "epilepsy" is employed. However, if a convulsive seizure is caused by a high dose of lidocaine, for example, the term "epilepsy" would be inappropriate.[3]

Seizures result from the rapid, excessive discharges of localized neural tissue often called "seizure foci." This rapid neural discharge may then spread throughout the central and the peripheral nervous systems. Anticonvulsant drugs produce a significant portion of their therapeutic effect by depressing the neurons which surround these seizure foci, thus preventing the spread of these excessive discharges.

Phenytoin (Dilantin) is the most widely used agent to prevent epileptic seizures. While there are many forms of epileptic seizures, petit mal is the only type that is not responsive to this drug. A noteworthy side effect which occurs in approximately 20 percent of patients taking phenytoin on a chronic basis is gingival hyperplasia. In this condition, the gums (gingiva) become enlarged and, in the more severe forms, actually cover the crowns of erupted teeth. The drug appears to sensitize the gingival tissues to local irritants, such as plaque and calculus (tartar), making rigid oral hygiene habits of paramount importance to patients taking this medication.[4]

Phenobarbital is the most widely employed barbiturate derivative since it is able to exert its anticonvulsive properties at doses lower than those required for its hypnotic effects. It is useful in all forms of epileptic seizures, but is most widely used alone or in combination with phenytoin for the prophylaxis of grand-mal–type episodes.

Most convulsive seizures are relatively brief in duration—less than five minutes. However, continuous convulsive episodes, such as status epilepticus or drug-induced seizures, pose a life-threatening condition that must be terminated pharmacologically. While phenytoin and barbiturates may be used, diazepam is considered the agent of choice based on its anticonvulsant efficacy and low incidence of respiratory depression. It is significant, however, that diazepam is not recommended as a prophylactic anticonvulsant because consistent anticonvulsant blood levels are difficult to maintain. Table 9.5 lists the popular anticonvulsant drugs and the type of seizures for which they are useful.

TABLE 9.5   Anticonvulsant preparations and seizure types for which they are effective

Preparation	Seizure type
phenytoin (Dilantin)	G, V
phenobarbital (Luminal)	G, V
carbamazepine (Tegretol)	G, V
ethosuximide (Zarontin)	P
trimethadione (Tridione)	P

G = grand mal   P = petit mal   V = various others

SYNOPSIS OF THERAPEUTIC AGENTS

I. **Sedative-hypnotic drugs**

   A. ACTION
     1. Depress neural discharge and/or potentiate the depressant action of inhibitory neurotransmitters, such as GABA

   B. USEFUL EFFECTS
     1. Calming (tranquilization)
     2. Sedation and hypnosis
     3. Anticonvulsant
     4. Skeletal muscle relaxation

   C. COMMON INDICATIONS
     1. Anxiety—preoperative or general
     2. Insomnia
     3. Seizures
     4. Skeletal muscle spasms

   D. PREPARATIONS
     1. Barbiturates—most likely to cause secondary effects
       a) Phenobarbital (Luminal)
     2. Benzodiazepines—least likely to cause secondary effects
       a) Diazepam (Valium)
     3. Antihistamines
       a) Hydroxyzine (Vistaril)

   E. SECONDARY EFFECTS
     1. Depress REM sleep
     2. Dependence
     3. Respiratory depression
     4. Cardiovascular depression
     5. Paradoxical CNS stimulation

II. **Anticonvulsants**

   A. ACTION
     1. Depress spread of impulses from irritable foci
     2. Depress irritable foci directly

   B. USEFUL EFFECTS
     1. Prevent seizure occurrence (prophylaxis)
     2. Terminate active seizure

   C. COMMON INDICATIONS
     1. All types of seizures—local and general

II. Anticonvulsants (*continued*)

D. PREPARATIONS
1. Grand mal prophylaxis
   a) Phenytoin (Dilantin)
   b) Phenobarbital (Luminal)
2. Petit mal
   a) Ethosuximide (Zarontin)
3. Status epilepticus
   a) Diazepam (Valium)
E. SECONDARY EFFECTS
1. Sedation
2. Gingival hyperplasia (only phenytoin)

ARTICLES FOR DISCUSSION

1. **Lundstrom, A., et al.** 1982. Effects of anti-epileptic drug treatment with carbamazepine or phenytoin on the oral state of children and adolescents. *Journal of Clinical Periodontology* 9:482–488.
2. **Tornetta, F. J.** 1977. A comparison of droperidol, diazepam, and hydroxyzine hydrochloride as premedication. *Anesthesia and Analgesia* 56:496–500.
3. **Safra, M. J., and Oakley, G. P.** 1975. Association between cleft lip with or without cleft palate and prenatal exposure to diazepam. Lancet 2:478–480.
4. **Rosenberg, L. et al.** 1983. Lack of relation of oral clefts to diazepam use during pregnancy. *New England Journal of Medicine* 309:1282–1285.
5. **Dominguez, R. A.** 1983. The benzodiazepines: A current review for the nonpsychiatrist. *Hospital Formulary* 18:1049–1056.
6. **Soloman, F., et al.** 1979. Sleeping pills, insomnia, and medical practice. *New England Journal of Medicine* 300:803.
7. **Dreifuss, F. E.** 1979. Use of anticonvulsant drugs. *JAMA* 241:607.
8. **Greenblatt, D. J., et al.** 1983. Current status of benzodiazepines. *New England Journal of Medicine* 309:354–8, 410–416.

REFERENCES

1. **Goodman, L. S., and Gilman, A.** 1980. *The Pharmacological Basis of Therapeutics*. 6th ed., New York: Macmillan, p. 352.

2. **Richter, J. J.** 1981. Current theories about the mechanisms of benzodiazepines and neuroleptic drugs. *Anesthesiology* 54:66–72.

3. **Goodman, L. S., and Gilman, A.** 1980. *The Pharmacological Basis of Therapeutics*. 6th ed. New York: Macmillan, pp. 448–450.

4. **Ciancio, S. G., et al.** 1972. Gingival hyperplasia and diphenylhydantoin. *Journal of Periodontology* 43:411.

10

Psychotropic Drugs

Drugs labeled "psychotropic" are those utilized to improve disorders in behavior. Typically they are subdivided into three categories, each representing the drug's primary indication. Antianxiety agents are those used to decrease anxiety, antipsychotic agents reduce psychotic symptoms, and finally, antidepressants are used to elevate depressive mood disorders. While some behavior syndromes may benefit from more than one therapeutic class, we will discuss each group separately.

ANTIANXIETY AGENTS

Drugs utilized to calm anxious or apprehensive patients are often referred to as anxiolytic drugs. In most cases, these agents are actually sedatives prescribed in subsedative doses. At these doses, patients quickly develop tolerance to any drowsiness while continuing to benefit from the calming effect, which itself probably represents a mild form of sedation. At the present time, the benzodiazepines are without rival in the treatment of anxiety.

> Some researchers have proposed a glycine-mimetic action by benzodiazepines in producing their anxiolytic effect. This discovery may eventually prove true for other sedative agents, and thereby disprove the above concept of antianxiety therapy.[1]

ANTIPSYCHOTIC AGENTS

Psychoses are those mental disorders in which the patient is unable to think coherently, comprehend reality, or even develop an awareness that a disorder exists. The biochemical mechanism producing this pathological state is poorly understood, but speculation concerning dopaminergic excess is tempting when one considers the mechanism of action of antipsychotic agents.

113

All antipsychotic agents improve psychotic behavior by virtue of blocking dopamine receptors within the cortex and the limbic system. Unfortunately they are not without numerous side effects including extrapyramidal effects, such as Parkinsonian tremors, orthostatic hypotension, and sedation. Very noteworthy, however, is their antiemetic efficacy making them extremely useful in treating nausea from most causes (chemotherapy, narcotics, motion sickness, and so forth).

The dopaminergic-receptor–blocking capability of antipsychotic agents accounts for many of their most noteworthy effects. The blockade of these receptors in the limbic regions and the cerebral cortex accounts for their antipsychotic effect, while the blockade of similar receptors in the chemotrigger zone (CTZ) of the medulla accounts for their antiemetic efficacy. Unfortunately, their ability to block dopaminergic activity in the basal ganglion mimics the dopamine-deficiency state seen in Parkinson's disease and thereby accounts for the many extrapyramidal symptoms displayed in patients taking these medications. While several categories of extrapyramidal symptoms may occur, tardive dyskinesia is particularly troublesome. It occurs following prolonged use of any antipsychotic agent and may actually worsen upon withdrawal of the offending agent. Typical involuntary motions include lip smacking and sucking, lateral jaw movements, and darting movements of the tongue. The pathogenesis is speculated to be excessive dopaminergic activity, which develops in an attempt to overcome the "antidopaminergic" action of the antipsychotic agents. Unlike other extrapyramidal symptoms, no effective therapy is available.

Antipsychotic drugs are also able to block alpha receptors on blood vessels leading to vasodilation and subsequent hypotension. Additionally, they are able to block cholinergic receptors, thereby producing many anticholinergic effects of which xerostomia (dry mouth) is most noteworthy. The dry oral mucous membrane facilitates ulcerations, erosions, and infection.

Several chemical classes of antipsychotic agents are available, but those derived from the phenothiazines are the most numerous. Chlorpromazine (Thorazine) is the prototype of the antipsychotic drugs and is very popular for both its antipsychotic and antiemetic effects. Table 10.1 lists the more popular agents, but one should keep in mind that the antipsychotic efficacy of these various preparations is quite comparable. However, there are notable differences in the type and the frequency of the side effects produced. Generally speaking, the more potent agents are most likely to produce extrapyramidal reactions and less likely to produce sedation and autonomic side effects. It is also important to remember that, despite their numerous side effects, the therapeutic index of most antipsychotic drugs is 200 or more.

TABLE 10.1 More commonly used antipsychotic agents*

Agents used to treat psychosis	Daily-dose range
chlorpromazine (Thorazine)	300–800 mg
thioridazine (Mellaril)	200–600 mg
mesoridazine (Serentil)	100–400 mg
triflupromazine (Vesprin)	50–150 mg
fluphenazine (Prolixin)	2.5–20 mg
thiothixene (Navane)	6–10 mg
trifluoperazine (Stelazine)	6–20 mg
haloperidol (Haldol)	6–20 mg
Agents used primarily as antiemetics	
promethazine (Phenergan)	
prochlorperazine (Compazine)	

*The more potent agents are less likely to produce sedation and autonomic side effects but more likely to produce extrapyramidal reactions.

ANTIDEPRESSANTS

Affective disorders are characterized by changes in mood, that is, mania and depression. Mania implies elation or hyperactivity and is generally treated with antipsychotic drugs. Depression, on the other hand, is treated with antidepressant drugs which elevate mood. Complicating the physician's selection is the fact that psychotic patients may also be depressed, in which case the choice between antipsychotic and antidepressant therapy is a challenging dilemma.

The antidepressants in use today, tricyclic antidepressants and monoamine oxidase inhibitors, were formerly thought to produce their mood-elevating effect by potentiating the action of norepinephrine and serotonin within the CNS. However, since this concept does not totally explain the efficacy of tricyclic compounds, central anticholinergic mechanisms as well as alterations in receptor populations may also play significant roles.

If we theorize that mental depression is a biogenic amine deficiency, drugs that inhibit monoamine oxidase (MAO inhibitors) and those that inhibit neuronal uptake mechanisms (tricyclic antidepressants) will prolong the action of CNS amines such as norepinephrine and serotonin. Unfortunately, the rapid onset of this action does not coincide with clinical improvement, which may not be observed for several weeks following the initiation of therapy.

The monoamine oxidase inhibitors (MAOI) are prescribed less frequently than the tricyclic compounds. They are generally not as effective and are associated with many toxic effects related to adverse interactions with foods and other drug preparations. Phenelzine (Nardil) is the most popular, but is generally used only when tricyclic antidepressants and electroconvulsive therapy (ECT) have proven ineffective. Recently there has been a rekindled interest in this drug class, but they have yet to regain their former status as "drugs of choice" for depressive disorders.

TABLE 10.2   Common antidepressant drugs

Tricyclic Compounds	Monoamine Oxidase Inhibitors (MAOI)
imipramine (Tofranil)	phenelzine (Nardil)
desipramine (Norpramin)	isocarboxazid (Marplan)
amitriptyline (Elavil)	tranylcypromine (Parnate)
nortriptyline (Aventyl)	
protriptyline (Vivactyl)	
doxepin (Sinequan)	

The tricyclic antidepressants are so named because of their three-ringed chemical configuration. There are six preparations in clinical use (Table 10.2), but imipramine (Tofranil) may be considered as the prototype of this group. There is no concrete evidence that any particular drug is more efficacious than others of this class. Their chemical structure is strikingly similar to that of the phenothiazine antipsychotic agents, and they share many of the side effects discussed in the previous section of this chapter.

The tricyclic compounds possess minimal antidopaminergic capability, producing only a small incidence of tremor, in contrast to the frequent extrapyramidal effects associated with the antipsychotic drugs. However, the tricyclic compounds do produce prominent anticholinergic side effects. Dry mouth, constipation, urinary retention, and blurred vision are frequently seen in patients maintained on tricyclic antidepressants.[2] This anticholinergic tendency combined with its primary action in potentiating adrenergic amines introduces the potential for serious cardiovascular consequences. Indeed, tachycardia, palpitations, and cardiac dysrhythmias have contributed to reports of myocardial infarction and heart failure associated with tricyclic therapy. Reported cases of intentional and accidental overdose, especially in children, have been increasing in the United States and present a major challenge to emergency-room physicians.[3,4]

It would be tempting to assume that tricyclic antidepressants are similar to stimulants such as amphetamines and therefore offer significant potential for abuse. However, this is not the case. Imipramine given to nondepressed patients produces sedation, light-headedness, and lethargy—none of which make it attractive for recreational use. Although similar effects are observed in depressed patients, elevation of mood develops following two to three weeks of therapy. This mood swing is more accurately described as a "dulling of depressive thinking" rather than a "euphoric stimulation" seen following amphetamine use. This effect pattern is so consistent that, following three weeks of therapy without improvement, a reevaluation of the original diagnosis is generally considered.

Despite the potential for side effects and overdose with these agents, the tricyclic antidepressants represent a dramatic improvement over former drug classes and remain the major therapeutic modality for treating depressive affective disorders.

SYNOPSIS OF THERAPEUTIC AGENTS

I. Antianxiety drugs (anxiolytic)

A. ACTION
1. Calm anxious and apprehensive symptoms by poorly defined mechanisms; it may represent a "subsedative" GABA-like action, or a totally different mechanism, for example, gylcine-mimetic

B. USEFUL EFFECTS
1. Calming (tranquilization)
2. Skeletal muscle relaxation

C. COMMON INDICATIONS
1. Anxiety
2. Preoperative
3. Skeletal muscle sasms

D. PREPARATIONS
1. Any benzodiazepine

E. SECONDARY EFFECTS
1. Same as sedative-hypnotics

II. Antipsychotic drugs

A. ACTION
1. Block dopamine receptors in limbic region

B. USEFUL EFFECTS
1. Improve psychotic symptoms
2. Antiemetic

C. COMMON INDICATIONS
1. Psychotic behavior
2. Nausea and vomiting

D. PREPARATIONS
1. Chlorpromazine (Thorazine)
2. Haloperidol (Haldol)

E. SECONDARY EFFECTS
1. Extrapyramidal symptoms
2. Orthostatic hypotension
3. Dry mouth

III. Tricyclic antidepressants

A. ACTION
  1. Inhibit reuptake of the biogenic amines, norepinephrine and serotonin
B. USEFUL EFFECT
  1. Suppress "depressive thinking"
C. COMMON INDICATIONS
  1. Depressive affective disorders
D. PREPARATIONS
  1. Imipramine (Tofranil)
  2. Amitriptyline (Elavil)
E. SECONDARY EFFECTS
  1. Sedation
  2. Cardiac dysrhythmia
  3. Any anticholinergic effect

ARTICLES FOR DISCUSSION

1. **Berry-Opersteny, D., and Heusinkveld, K. B.** 1983. Prophylactic antiemetics for chemotherapy-associated nausea and vomiting. *Cancer Nursing* 6:117–123.
2. **Reich, S. D.** 1983. Metoclopramide: A brief review. *Cancer Nursing* 6:71–73.
3. **Gralla, R. J. et al.** 1981. Antiemetic efficacy of high-dose metoclopramide: Randomized trials with placebo and prochlorperazine in patients with chemotherapy-induced nausea and vomiting. *New England Journal of Medicine* 305:905–909.
4. **Richter, J. J.** 1981. Current theories about the mechanisms of benzodiazepines and neuroleptic drugs. *Anesthesiology* 54:66–72.
5. **Thompson, T. L., et al.** 1983. Psychotropic drug use in the elderly. *New England Journal of Medicine* 308:134–138, 194–198.
6. **Rosal-Greif, V. F.** 1982. Drug-induced dyskinesias. *American Journal of Nursing* 82:66–69.
7. **Baptista, R. S.** 1981. The tricyclic antidepressants: A Current Perspective. *Hospital Formulary* 16:724.
8. **Greenblatt, D. J. et al.** 1983. Current status of benzodiazepines. *New England Journal of Medicine* 309:354–358, 410–416.

REFERENCES

1. Iversen, L. L. Iversen, S. D., and Snyder, S. H. 1978. *Handbook of Psychopharmacology,* Vol. 10. New York: Plenum Press.

2. Blackwell, B., et al. 1978. Anticholinergic activity of two tricyclic antidepressants. *American Journal of Psychiatry* 135:722–724.

3. Boston Collaborative Drug Surveillance Program. 1972. Adverse reactions to tricyclic antidepressant drugs. *Lancet* 1:529–530.

4. Williams, R. B., and Sherter, C. 1971. Cardiac complications of tricyclic antidepressant therapy. *Annals of Internal Medicine* 74:395–398.

11

Analgesic Preparations

It would be difficult to imagine a health profession that does not deal with the patient experiencing pain. More than any topic in this text, analgesics require familiarity by all health care professionals. To better appreciate the rationale for analgesic selection, we must grasp basic concepts of pain transmission.

THE PAIN PATHWAY

Following any tissue injury, chemicals are synthesized and/or released by the damaged cells. These so-called "pain mediators" stimulate sensory nerve endings, which results in an impulse conducted towards the central nervous system. Prostaglandins are a class of compounds which appear to sensitize the nerve endings to pain mediators such as bradykinin. Prostaglandin synthesis inhibitors, such as aspirin, are therefore able to reduce the pain experience at its source.

Once the sensory fiber has been stimulated, the impulse is conducted into the spinal cord where the nerve fiber synapses with many intermediate neurons within a region of the dorsal horn called the substantia gelatinosa. From this region, fibers cross to the opposite side of the cord and ascend to the brain within the lateral spinothalamic tracts. In the thalamus, the impulse is relayed to many other brain regions, such as the cortex and the limbic regions (see Figure 11.1).

It is possible to interfere with this pathway by utilizing four basic classes of pharmacological agents. Aspirin-like agents lessen the effect of the initial stimulus while local anesthetics block conduction of the impulse along the sensory nerves. Once the impulse has entered the central nervous system, narcotic analgesics and general anesthetics are able to depress the perception of the impulse.

In contrast to anesthetics, which depress all sensory perception, such as

121

pain, temperature, and pressure, the analgesics are drugs which reduce only the sensation of pain. These agents may be classified conveniently as either narcotic or non-narcotic analgesics. The former are those resembling morphine which exert their action centrally within the brain or the spinal cord. The latter agents resemble aspirin and produce their action peripherally at the site of tissue injury.

Figure 11.1 The pain pathway illustrating the site of action of various analgesic modalities.

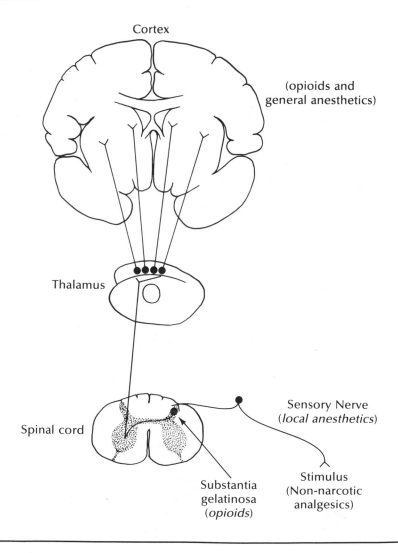

NON-NARCOTIC ANALGESICS

The non-narcotic analgesics include acetaminophen (Tylenol), aspirin, and other agents resembling aspirin in action and effects. All the non-narcotic drugs inhibit the synthesis of prostaglandins and thereby reduce the stimulation of sensory nerve endings by pain mediators. Since the prostaglandins perform many functions, including fever production and inflammation, it is not surprising that this class of drugs also possesses antipyretic and, with the exception of acetaminophen, anti-inflammatory efficacy.

Now that the three primary effects have been established, let us consider secondary effects of our prototype, aspirin. The most conspicuous side effects relate to the gastrointestinal tract and include irritation, nausea, and vomiting. Since aspirin is quite acidic, you may well imagine its irritating properties to skin and mucous membranes. Severe ulcerations and erosions are seen when patients place an aspirin tablet on a tooth as a toothache remedy. Although not so visible, this same mucosal effect can occur throughout the GI tract. Even one day of aspirin therapy has been viewed endoscopically to produce mild degrees of GI bleeding and ulceration.[1]

> The gastrointestinal effects of aspirin are not totally due to a direct irritant "mechanism." There is evidence that certain species of prostaglandins may be protective to GI mucosa by virtue of stimulating protective mucous production. By inhibiting the synthesis of these "protective" prostaglandins, gastric erosion is facilitated. This would explain the similar GI effects produced by aspirinlike agents which are not directly irritating to mucous membranes.[2]

It is surprising that most people tolerate these GI effects and seldom suffer clinically significant mucosal damage. Obviously those patients already suffering GI disturbances, such as peptic ulcer, should avoid an aspirinlike preparation.

Aspirin inhibits platelet aggregation by inhibiting the formation of thromboxane, a metabolite in the prostaglandin pathway. The resulting anticoagulant effect, combined with its erosive potential, contra-indicates its use in patients undergoing anticoagulant therapy, for example, Coumadin.

> Recent studies show that this platelet effect is benefical for patients prone towards coronary artery disease. Low doses, less than 300 mg/day, produce blood levels sufficient to inhibit synthesis of thromboxane A_2, one of the mediators of platelet aggregation. This low dose does not appear to inhibit prostacyclin and prostaglandin synthesis, thus permitting their normal physiological roles to continue.[3,4]

Hypersensitivity (allergy) or asthmatic reactions to aspirin are not uncommon and represent an obvious contraindication. Since cross-hypersensitivity occurs with other aspirinlike preparations, they should be withheld from patients claiming allergy to aspirin. Indeed, many patients suffering apparent allergic reactions to zomepirac (subsequently withdrawn from the market) were also documented as hypersensitive to aspirin.

It is doubtful that the mechanism responsible for hypersensitivity is truly immunological in nature, since cross-hypersensitivity occurs between aspirinlike drugs which are structurally dissimilar. Cross-hypersensitivity is especially prevalent with those agents expressly effective in inhibiting the E series of prostaglandins, which normally protect against inflammatory mediator release. Thus, blocking the synthesis of protective prostaglandins facilitates mediator release and subsequent "allergic-like" symptoms.[5]

In addition to the above adverse effects, chronic aspirin overdose presents a series of symptoms collectively referred to as "salicylism." In addition to severe gastrointestinal disturbances, these symptoms include headache, tinnitus, hyperthermia, and hyperventilation. Treatment consists of supportive measures along with sodium bicarbonate administration to correct acidosis.

Acetaminophen (Tylenol) is a non-narcotic analgesic that differs from aspirinlike drugs in several manners. While equal to aspirin in relieving pain and fever, it lacks any significant anti-inflammatory efficacy. For this reason, it is useful for treating pain but not inflammation associated with arthritis. Its ability to inhibit prostaglandin synthesis is more notable centrally than in peripheral tissues and may eventually be proven to exert its total therapeutic effect at CNS locations. However, it does not interact with opioid receptors and will therefore retain its classification as a "non-narcotic" analgesic.

Acetaminophen lacks any aspirinlike adverse effects on the GI tract or platelets and demonstrates no cross-hypersensitivity to these preparations. For these reasons it is the logical alternative when aspirin is contra-indicated. However, one must not assume it to be without adverse effects. Acute doses exceeding 15 grams (in adults weighing 70 kg) will lead to severe hepatotoxicity and is not an unusual occurrence, especially when one considers the cavalier attitude given most over-the-counter preparations.

It is a metabolite of acetaminophen, rather than the parent compound, that induces hepatic necrosis. This toxic metabolite is normally conjugated with glutathione and transported for renal excretion. However, when an acute dose exceeds the amount of glutathione available, the metabolite accumulates in the liver. Treatment consists of high oral doses of N-acetyl-cysteine (Mucomyst) which replaces glutathione stores, thus removing the toxic metabolite.[6]

Aspirin and acetaminophen are equally potent and efficacious in reducing both fever and pain. Their optimal analgesic dose is typically quoted to be 650 mg, but newer studies support a positive dose-response to continue up to 1000 mg.[7] Most clinical studies have demonstrated slightly superior analgesic efficacy with other non-narcotic preparations.[8,9] Table 11.1 lists some of the more popular agents available. The anti-inflammatory properties of these agents will be addressed in Chapter 15. Most critical is the fact that, excluding acetaminophen, a contraindication for aspirin must be considered a contraindication for any of these.

TABLE 11.1 Nonnarcotic agents utilized as analgesics*

aspirin (Bayer, et al.)	ibuprofen (Motrin)
acetaminophen (Tylenol et al.)	fenoprofen (Nalfon)
diflunisal (Dolobid)	naproxen (Naprosyn)
mefenamic acid (Ponstel)	

---

*Excluding acetaminophen, these agents may also be prescribed as anti-inflammatory agents and will be discussed in Chapter 15.
**Now available OTC as Nuprin and Advil.

NARCOTIC ANALGESICS

Narcotics are those analgesics which resemble opium in action. For this reason it is common to refer to them as "opioids" and to the receptors with which they react as "opioid receptors." These receptors were identified in 1973[10] stimulating the search for the endogenous substance (ligand) with which they interact. (Given the unlikelihood that our "maker" would endow us with a receptor for heroin!) By 1976, the endogenous compounds were identified and assigned the names, enkephalin and endorphin. Subsequently, numerous additional ligands have been identified, synthesized, and classified as enkephalins or endorphins.

All endogenous opioids are peptides in structure, ranging from the pentapeptide enkephalins to the 31 amino acid sequence of beta-endorphin. The former compounds are thought to function as neurotransmitters while the polypeptides function as hormones. ALL of the significant amino acid sequences, as well as that of ACTH, are contained in the pituitary hormone aptly named, preopiocortin.

The normal physiological roles of these ligands is unsettled, but convincing evidence supports their role in pain tolerance[11], placebo[12], and acupuncture[13].

The prototype of the narcotic analgesics is morphine, which occurs naturally in the opium extracted from the pods of the poppy plant. Many of the popular opioid analgesics are semi-synthetic derivatives of morphine and differ mainly in potency, efficacy, and frequency of adverse effects, including abuse potential.

TABLE 11.2   Secondary effects produced by morphine and most other opioids

sedation	dependence	constipation
respiratory depression	miotic pupils	histamine release
hypotension		nausea and vomiting

Heroin, diacetylmorphine, owes most of its actual effects to the morphine molecule to which it is biotransformed in the liver. Although originally heralded as a "heroic" analgesic by the Bayer company, its rapid passage through the blood-brain barrier accounts for a "euphoric rush" following intravenous administration. Its proven abuse potential and lack of superior efficacy to morphine make any future legalization in the USA unlikely.[14]

Morphine produces virtually all of its CNS and gastrointestinal effects by activity as an opioid-receptor agonist. Its primary use is for the relief of severe pain where less efficacious agents have failed. Its secondary effects are shared, more or less, by most of the opioid preparations and are listed in Table 11.2. Of greatest concern is its ability to depress CO_2 sensitivity in medullary neurons. The ensuing respiratory depression is invariably the cause of death from any opioid overdose. Tolerance to this, as well as many of the other effects, occurs consistently and accounts for the very large doses used by narcotic addicts. Of interest is the fact that miotic and constipating tolerances do not occur. One result is that the addict is condemned to stumbling, night-time strolls to the emergency room for fecal impaction removal. Table 11.3 lists the popular opioid agonists and their potencies relative to morphine.

TABLE 11.3 Opioid agonists with doses required to produce comparable effects to 10 mg of morphine

Opioid agonist	Equivalent Dose
diacetylmorphine (Heroin)	3 mg
hydromorphone (Dilaudid)	1.5 mg
oxymorphone (Numorphan)	1 mg
levorphanol (Levo-Dromoran)	3mg
methadone (Dolophine)	10 mg
meperidine (Demerol)	100 mg
codeine*	120 mg
proproxyphene (Darvon)*	130 mg

*Comparable analgesic efficacy to morphine is questionable even at this dose. Nausea and constipation generally limit the use of this or higher doses.

Several species of opioid receptors have been proposed, each accounting for different narcotic effects (see Table 11.4). Because analgesia can be produced by receptors that do not produce dependence, it seems possible to synthesize agents that lack affinity for the mu receptor.

TABLE 11.4 Putative opioid receptors and their different narcotic effects*

Mu Receptors:	Kappa Receptors:	Sigma Receptors:
supraspinal analgesia	spinal analgesia	dysphoria
respiratory depression	miosis	hallucinations
euphoria	sedation	respiratory and vaso-motor stimulation
dependence		

*Additional subspecies of receptors are presently being researched.

Presently there are three such agents which act as antagonists on the mu receptors but as agonists on the kappa and sigma sites (see Table 11.5). It would follow that these agents should be less likely to produce physical dependence and respiratory depression. Although less than perfect in reality, they have been shown to produce withdrawal in patients dependent on morphine or heroin. With this in mind, it is prudent to avoid their use in chronic-pain patients where dependence to morphine or meperidine is likely. These agents are quite popular as analgesics for obstetrical cases and myocardial infarction where avoidance of respiratory depression is critical.

In myocardial infarction, morphine is used not only for its analgesic and calming effects, but for its hemodynamic properties. While decreased peripheral resistance leads to hypotension, it is beneficial to the ischemic myocardium since it leads to a reduction in work effort (reduced preload and afterload). Studies have shown nalbuphine comparable to morphine in this regard while producing less respiratory depression.[15,16]

TABLE 11.5 Agonist-antagonist opioids presently available in the United States

Opioid	Brand Name
pentazocine	Talwin
butorphanol	Stadol
nalbuphine	Nubain

Naloxone (Narcan) is the only narcotic antagonist in routine clinical use. It rapidly reverses all narcotic effects within minutes following intravenous injection. It accomplishes this dramatic effect by displacing opioid agonists from their receptors, but its effect may not exceed the half-life of longer-acting opioids, such as morphine, necessitating additional doses. Naloxone is generally considered innocuous and is often included in standing orders for the treatment of any patient apneic from unknown causes.

Since naloxone also blocks the receptor affinity of enkephalins and endorphins, the normal physiological roles of these endogenous peptides are also reversed. This may warrant reevaluation of naloxone's proposed "innocuous behavior."

It appears that some of the endogenous opioids play a role in depressing sympathoadrenal stimulation of the cardiovascular system. By blocking this protective effect, naloxone may precipitate cardiovascular stimulation. This may account for the scattered reports of sudden death following naloxone administration.[17] Of equal significance is naloxone's potential in the treatment of hypotension and shock. Dramatic recoveries have been attributed to naloxone after pressor agents have failed to reverse the shock syndrome in selected patients.[18,19]

COMBINATION PRODUCTS

The most widely prescribed analgesic products are compounds containing either aspirin or acetaminophen combined with codeine or a derivative. They offer the advantage of interrupting the pain pathway peripherally as well as centrally. This synergistic analgesic effect lessens the amount of narcotic required, which is of obvious benefit.

Compounds are typically numbered, for example, Tylenol #3, with the number representing the amount of codeine present: #1 = 7.5 mg, #2 = 15 mg, #3 = 30 mg, and #4 = 60 mg. Products containing codeine derivatives do not use this numbering system. Table 11.6 lists some of the more popular products, and one should not assume any pharmacological uniqueness to any specific preparation. If you grasp the actions and the effects of aspirin, acetaminophen, and opioids, then you understand any of these combination products. Because many patients cannot tolerate aspirin, its presence in any compound should be ascertained before administering these agents to your patients.

TABLE 11.6 Commonly prescribed analgesic combination products

Brand Name	Major Ingredients
Empirin #1–4	aspirin and codeine
Tylenol #1–4	acetaminophen codeine
Percodan	aspirin and oxycodone
Tylox	acetaminophen and oxycodone
Darvon Compound	aspirin, phenacetin, caffeine, and propoxyphene
Darvocet-N 100	acetaminophen and propoxyphene

The inclusion of caffeine in various aspirin and acetaminophen combinations has been criticized for quite some time. This criticism is quite understandable considering the lack of valid clinical studies demonstrating the superior efficacy of this combination over aspirin or acetaminophen alone. Although the superior efficacy of this combination has not been proven, recent analysis of clinical studies does support the fact that caffeine increases the potency of aspirin and acetaminophen. In other words, the inclusion of caffeine enables a lower dose of aspirin or acetaminophen to produce the same analgesic effect as that produced by either of these analgesics alone.[20]

The role of analgesic adjuvants is gaining widespread credibility in treating patients suffering various chronic pain syndromes. Amphetamines, antipsychotics, anxiolytics, and antidepressants have all demonstrated efficacy in potentiating the analgesic effect of opioid agonists. The exact mechanism of this positive effect is not established, but certainly their alteration of neurotransmitter functions within the limbic structures is an attractive hypothesis.[21,22]

SYNOPSIS OF THERAPEUTIC AGENTS

I. Aspirin-like analgesics

A. ACTION
   1. Inhibit synthesis of prostaglandins, thereby preventing their ability to induce pain, fever, and inflammation
B. USEFUL EFFECTS
   1. Analgesia
   2. Antipyretic
   3. Anti-inflammatory
C. COMMON INDICATIONS
   1. Pain
   2. Fever
   3. Inflammation
D. PREPARATIONS
   1. Aspirin
   2. Ibuprofen (Motrin)
E. SECONDARY EFFECTS
   1. Gastrointestinal disturbances
      a) Bleeding
      b) Irritation
      c) Nausea and vomiting
   2. Inhibit platelet aggregation
   3. Hypersensitivity

II. Acetaminophen

A. COMPARED TO ASPIRIN
   1. Same mechanism of action
   2. Lacks anti-inflammatory efficacy
   3. Lacks secondary effects of aspirin
      a) Hepatotoxicity in high doses

III. Opioids

A. ACTION
   1. Interact with opioid receptors
B. USEFUL EFFECTS
   1. Analgesia
   2. Sedation (may be undesirable)
   3. Antitussive
   4. Antidiarrheal (may be undesirable)

III. Opioids *(continued)*

    E. SECONDARY EFFECTS
- 1. Respiratory depression
- 2. Hypotension
- 3. Dependence
- 4. Nausea and vomiting

    C. COMMON INDICATIONS
- 1. Pain
- 2. Severe diarrhea
- 3. To suppress cough

    D. PREPARATIONS
- 1. Morphine
- 2. Meperidine (Demerol)
- 3. Codeine

    E. SECONDARY EFFECTS
- 1. Respiratory depression
- 2. Hypotension
- 3. Dependence
- 4. Nausea and vomiting

ARTICLES FOR DISCUSSION

1. **Simon, L. J., and Mills, J. A.** 1980. Nonsteroidal anti-inflammatory drugs. *New England Journal of Medicine* 302:1179–1185, 1237–1242.
2. **Crossley, H. L., et al.** 1983. Nonsteroidal anti-inflammatory agents in relieving dental pain: A Review. *Journal of the American Dental Association* 106:61–64.
3. **Dingfelder, J. R.** 1981. Primary dysmenorrhea treatment with prostaglandin inhibitors: A Review. *American Journal of Obstetrics and Gynecology* 140:874–879.
4. **Rumack, B. H., et al.** 1981. Acetaminophen overdose: Six hundred sixty-two cases with evaluation of oral acetylcysteine treatment. *Archives of Internal Medicine* 141:380–385.
5. **Becker, D. E.** 1982. Synopsis of endogenous opiate research. *Dental Hygiene* 56:38–40.

6. **Kaiko, R. F., et al.** 1981. Analgesic and mood effects of heroin and morphine in cancer patients with postoperative pain. *New England Journal of Medicine* 304:1501–1505.

7. **Wescoe, G. W.** 1980. The Brompton cocktail, no more effective than oral narcotic analgesics in chronic pain. *Hospital Formulary* p. 266–268; editorial, p. 328.

8. **Rankin, M. A.** 1982. Use of drugs for pain with cancer patients. *Cancer Nursing* 5:181–190.

9. **Bishop, B.** 1980. Pain: Its physiology and rationale for management. *Physical Therapy* 60:13–37.

10. **Cooper, S. A. et al.** 1980. Evaluation of oxycodone and acetaminophen in the treatment of postoperative dental pain. *Oral Surgery* 50:496–502.

REFERENCES

1. **Hoftiezer, J. W., et al.** 1982. Effects of 24 Hours of aspirin, Bufferin, paracetamol and placebo on normal human gastrointestinal mucosa. *GUT* 23:692–697.

2. **Goodman, L. S., and Gilman, A.** 1980. *The Pharmacological Basis of Therapeutics*. 6th ed. New York: Macmillan, pp. 686–691.

3. **Lewis, D. H., et al.** 1983. Protective effects of aspirin against acute myocardial infarction and death in men with unstable angina. *New England Journal of Medicine* 309:396–403.

4. **Moncada, S., and Vane, J. R.** 1979. Arachidonic acid metabolites and the interactions between platelets and blood vessel walls. *New England Journal of Medicine* 300:1142–1147.

5. **Sczeklik, A., et al.** 1977. Clinical patterns of hypersensitivity to nonsteroidal anti-inflammatory drugs and their pathogenesis. *Journal of Allergy and Clinical Immunology* 60:276–284.

6. **Georgetown University Symposium.** 1981. Aspirin and acetaminophen. *Archives of Internal Medicine* 41:375–389.

7. **Cooper, S. A. et al.** 1980. Evaluation of oxycodone and acetaminophen in the treatment of postoperative dental pain. *Oral Surgery* 50:496–502.

8. **Forbes, J. A., et al.** 1982. Diflunisal. *JAMA* 248:2139–2142.

9. **Cooper, S. A. et al.** 1977. Comparative analgesic potency of aspirin and ibuprofen. *Journal of Oral Surgery* 35:898–903.

10. **Pert, C. B., and Snyder, S. H.** 1973. Opiate receptor: Demonstration in nervous tissue. *Science* 179:1011–1014.

11. Bortz, W., et al. 1981. Catecholamines, dopamine, and endorphin levels during extreme exercise. *New England Journal of Medicine* 305:466–467.

12. Levine, J. D., et al. 1978. The mechanism of placebo analgesia. *Lancet* 2:654–658.

13. Pomeranz, G., and Chiu, D. 1976. Naloxone blockage of acupuncture analgesia: Endorphin implicated. *Life Sciences* 19:1757–1762.

14. Kaiko, R. F., et al. 1981. Analgesic and mood effects of heroin and morphine in cancer patients with postoperative pain. *New England Journal of Medicine* 304:1501–1555.

15. Lee, G., et al. 1981. Hemodynamic effects of morphine and nalbuphine in acute myocardial infarction. *Clinical Pharmacology and Therapeutics* 29:576–581.

16. Gal, et al. 1982. Analgesic and respiratory depressant activity of nalbuphine: A comparison with morphine. *Anesthesiology* 57:367–374.

17. Andree, R. A. 1980. Sudden death following naloxone administration. *Anesthesia and Analgesia* 59:782.

18. Higgins, T. L., et al. 1983. Reversal of hypotension by continuous naloxone infusion in a ventilator-dependent patient. *Annals of Internal Medicine* 98:47–48.

19. Dzierba, S. H., and Latiolais, C. J. 1983. Naloxone reversal of hypotension and the shock syndrome. *Hospital Formulary* 18:723–728.

20. Laska, E. M., et al. 1984. Caffeine as an analgesic adjuvant. *JAMA* 251:1711–1718.

21. Fields, H. L. 1981. Pain. II: New approaches to management. *Annals of Neurology* 9:101–106.

22. Boukoons, A. J. 1981. Analgesic adjuvants: The role of psychotropics, anticonvulsants, and prostaglandin inhibitors. *Drug Therapy (hospital edition)* 41–48.

12

General Anesthesia

It is startling to imagine having to undergo a surgical procedure without being anesthetized. Yet this was always so prior to William T.G. Morton's now famous demonstration of ether anesthesia at Massachusetts General Hospital in 1846.

> With Horace Wells's failure in nitrous oxide anesthesia firmly established, observers at this demonstration were quite skeptical. But following the successful induction with ether, the surgeon, Dr. Warren, turned to the gallery of observers and said, "Gentlemen, this is no humbug." Another surgeon in attendance said of Dr. Morton's demonstration, "I have seen something today that will go around the world."

Appropriately, the following epitaph may be found on Dr. Morton's monument in Boston:

> *Inventor and revealer of anesthetic inhalation*
> *Before whom, in all time, surgery was agony*
> *By whom pain in surgery was averted and annulled*
> *Since whom science has control of pain.*

Today ether anesthesia has been entirely replaced by agents safer and more rapid in onset. Although Guedel's classical stages of ether anesthesia are no longer witnessed, one can use them to conceptualize the progression from consciousness to a state of general anesthesia.

Stage I—Analgesia: The patient becomes sedated and develops a mild analgesic state wherein he or she is not so responsive to mild pain stimuli. Today, this stage actually commences following preoperative medication and, in itself, may serve as an adequate depth for procedures performed under local anesthesia, such as dental surgery or arthroscopy.

Stage II—Delirium: As the patient loses consciousness, a classic fight-or-flight response occurs, witnessed as an increase in respiratory rate, heart rate, and blood pressure, as well as in retching. Since the more contemporary agents induce anesthesia in the patient so rapidly, this stage is fortunately avoided.

Stage III—Surgical Anesthesia: In this stage, vital signs return to normal and CNS functions are depressed progressively until adequate surgical depth is achieved. Various levels of depth within this stage may be described as planes 1 through 4 and are delineated by the progressive loss of reflexes and skeletal muscle tone (see Table 12.1). Simultaneously respiratory and cardiovascular functions deteriorate until total medullary paralysis occurs (Stage IV). Let us hope that this last stage is of academic interest only!

Anesthetists and anesthesiologists interpret anesthetic depth by monitoring vital signs, muscle tone (assuming absence of muscle relaxants), and reflexive responses to the surgeon's procedures.

ANESTHETIC MECHANISMS

Many theories have been advanced to explain the mechanism by which general anesthesia is produced, but none are conclusive. A major dilemma results from the dissimilar molecular structures of the many agents capable of inducing a general anesthetic state. This, of course, renders a receptor mechanism unlikely. Most acceptable are putative mechanisms which render reticular neuronal membranes incapable of the conformational changes required for impulse conduction and neurotransmitter release.[1]

Anesthetic agents are easily categorized according to their route of administration: inhalation and intravenous. Although specific regimens may vary considerably, in general, patients are induced with intravenous agents and then maintained at the desired anesthetic depth with a combination of inhalation and intravenous agents.

INHALATION ANESTHETICS

The anesthetic gases are fairly comparable in anesthetic efficacy but vary in potency and nature of secondary effects. The issue of potency is not so easily ascertained as it is with liquids or solids which use units of weight, for example, milligrams. With this in mind, anesthesiologists have adopted the concept of minimum alveolar concentration (MAC) as a method for comparing anesthetic potency. The MAC of a gas is the percentage of concentration of the gas in the alveoli that is required to render 50 percent of the patients unresponsive to surgical stimulation. This may be likened to the ED_{50} described in Chapter 1 of

TABLE 12.1 Guedel's scheme of progressive CNS depression produced by the anesthetic ether. Changes in physiologic functions are shown for the different stages and planes of Guedel's classification. Examples of surgery that can be performed at these anesthetic levels are given in parentheses.

Stage: plane	Respiration — Intercostal	Respiration — Diaphragm	Blood pressure and pulse	Reflexes — Pharyngeal laryngeal	Reflexes — Ocular	Pupil size	Muscle tone
Stage I: Analgesia (dental surgery)							
Stage II: Delirium (no surgery)				Swallow Retch Vomit	Lid		
Stage III: Plane 1 (dental and thoracic surgery)					Conjunctival		
Plane 2 (abdominal surgery)					Corneal		
Plane 3 (deep abdominal surgery)				Laryngeal Bronchial	Pupil light reflex		
Plane 4 (no surgery)							
Stage IV: Medullary paralysis → Death							

Reprinted with permission from Neidle, E. A. et al. 1980. *Pharmacology and Therapeutics for Dentistry*. St. Louis, C. V. Mosby.

course. From information in Table 12.2, one can deduce a phenomenal difference in potency between the fluorinated hydrocarbons and nitrous oxide. Whereas anesthesia may be induced and maintained with only a 2 percent concentration of these agents, it requires a 105 percent concentration of nitrous oxide. The minimum oxygen requirement of 20 to 30 percent obviously precludes the use of nitrous oxide as a single anesthetic agent, since the maximum percent one could safely deliver is 70 to 80 percent! Despite this lack of potency, its analgesic properties and relative lack of toxic effects makes it a very popular adjuvant with other inhalation and intravenous agents. Its presence in the anesthetic regime permits a reduction in the concentration of other gases, that is, lowered MAC, thereby reducing the likelihood of anesthetic toxicity. Aside from this, nitrous oxide in concentrations of 20 to 50 percent provides sedation and analgesia useful for conscious dental and obstetrical procedures.

Since most of the inhalation anesthetics possess comparable anesthetic efficacy, they are generally compared according to their adverse effects on cardiac function, blood pressure, and liver toxicity (see Table 12.2).

TABLE 12.2 Comparison of potencies and adverse effects of inhalation general anesthetics

	MAC	Reduced Cardiac Output	Hypotension	Cardiac Irritability	Liver Toxicity
Halothane (Fluothane)	.75	+ +	+ +	+ +	+ +
Methoxyflurane* (Penthrane)	.16	+ +	+	+	+
Enflurane (Ethrane)	1.68	+ +	+	+	+
Isoflurane (Forane)	1.40	0	+	0	0 (+ ?)
Nitrous oxide	105.00	0	0	0	0

+ = mild
+ + = significant
*Very limited use as a result of renal toxicity from high plasma fluoride levels.

INTRAVENOUS ANESTHETICS

Ultrashort-acting barbiturates are the most popular agents for inducing the general anesthetic state. The onset of unconsciousness is smooth and rapid (10 to 20 seconds) following an intravenous bolus. Since the depression of cardiovascular and respiratory function is more pronounced with barbiturates than inhalation agents, they are not attractive as sole anesthetic agents for prolonged procedures. It is typical to supplement these agents with intravenous opioids, neuroleptics, and inhalation agents, a procedure popularly referred to as "balanced anesthesia." Thiopental sodium (Pentothal) and methohexital (Brevital) are commonly used preparations and may be administered by either intermittent boluses or continuous drip either for induction or throughout the duration of the surgical procedure.

Various combinations of opioids and tranquilizing agents may be included in the anesthetic regime, a procedure commonly described as "neurolept anesthesia." Most popular is the combination of fentanyl and droperidol, marketed as Innovar. Such neuroleptic regimes may be employed alone for minor surgery and diagnostic procedures or in combination with barbiturates and inhalation agents during a balanced anesthesia technique.

Ketamine (Ketalar) is a unique anesthetic which is described as producing a "disassociative" form of anesthesia. It produces a light stage of anesthesia in which a patient experiences analgesia and disassociation from the environment. Ketamine's site of action appears to involve cortical and limbic regions rather than the reticular formation typical of other anesthetics.[2] For this reason, unpleasant dreams and hallucinations may occur during recovery and require that a quiet postoperative environment be available during recovery. Airway reflexes and respiratory function are not depressed by ketamine. This property offers a unique advantage in changing burn dressings, especially those about the head and the neck.

PREOPERATIVE MEDICATION

The goals of preoperative medications are sedation, analgesia, drying of oropharyngeal secretions, and prevention of vagal reflexes, such as bradycardia. Virtually any sedative or narcotic will fulfill the first two goals, while anticholinergic agents provide the final objectives. The more popular agents used in preoperative regimens are listed in Table 12.3. These medications may be administered PO, IV, or IM, with the latter route being most typical.

TABLE 12.3 Sedative, narcotic, and anticholinergic agents utilized for preoperative medication

Narcotics	Sedatives	Anticholinergics
morphine	diazepam (Valium)	atropine
meperidine (Demerol)	lorazepam (Ativan)	scopolamine
oxymorphone (Numorphan)	pentobarbital (Nembutal)	glycopyrrolate (Robinul)
	hydroxyzine (Vistaril)	

SYNOPSIS OF THERAPEUTIC AGENTS

The following synopsis consists of a typical general anesthetic sequence. One must keep in mind that the exact drug selection and dosage vary with the patient and medical status.

I. **Preoperative medication** (administered one hour before surgery IM)

  A. meperidine, (Demerol) 50 mg
  B. hydroxyzine (Vistaril), 25 mg
  C. atropine, .4 mg

II. **Patient transported to operating room**

  A. I.V. established; while awaiting surgeon, 1 ml Innovar IV (containing 0.05 mg fentanyl and 2.5 mg droperidol)
  B. Patient breathing 100 percent O_2
  C. Induction with 50 to 100 mg increments of Pentothal
  D. Patient breathing 60 percent N_2O and 40% O_2
  E. Succinylcholine 70 to 100 mg IV for muscle relaxation prior to tracheal intubation
  F. Patient breathing 1 percent Ethrane, 60 percent N_2O, and 39 percent O_2 (with additional increments of Pentothal and/or Innovar as necessary to maintain anesthetic depth)

ARTICLES FOR DISCUSSION

1. **Forrest, W. H., et al.** 1977. Subjective responses to six common preoperative medications. *Anesthesiology* 47:241–247.
2. **Tornetta, F. J.** 1977. Comparison of droperidol, diazepam, and hydroxyzine hydrochloride as premedication. *Anesthesia and Analgesia* 56:496–500.
3. **Hovi-Viander M., et al.** 1980. A comparative study of the clinical effects of Pentobarbital and diazepam given orally as preoperative medication. *Journal of Oral Surgery* 38:188–190.
4. **Leonard, L.** 1981. General principles of anesthesia. *Surgical Technologist* 13:26–30.
5. **Hornbein, R. F., et al.** 1982. Minimum alveolar concentration of nitrous oxide in man. *Anesthesia and Analgesia* 61:553–556.
6. **Wade, J. G., and Stevens, W. C.** 1981. Isoflurane—An anesthetic for the '80s? *Anesthesia and Analgesia* 60:666–682.

REFERENCES

1. Trudell, J. R. 1977. A unitary theory of anesthesia based on lateral phase separations in nerve membranes. *Anesthesiology* 46:5–10.

2. Winters, W. D., et al. 1972. The cataleptic state induced by ketamine: A review of the neuropharmacology of anesthesia. *Neuropharmacology* 11:303–315.

13

Endocrine Function

The endocrine system is a collection of organs which release their products into the bloodstream, thereby differing from their exocrine counterparts, which release substances via duct systems. These endocrine secretions are called hormones and arrive at their destination (target organ), along with other vascular travelers such as oxygen and nutrients. All of the body's hormones may be structurally classified as either steroids or amino acid derivatives, for example, proteins.

> It is more accurate to subdivide hormones into "local" and "general" to accommodate neurohormones whose target organs are in proximity to the site of their release from neurons, such as norepinephrine and acetylcholine.
>
> There are two mechanisms by which hormones act on target tissues. The peptides interact with cell-membrane receptors, which results in altered membrane permeability or in the synthesis of a "second messenger" called cyclic AMP. This messenger then produces the different physiological effects. The steroidal hormones interact with receptors within the cytoplasm, which leads to the synthesis of proteins. These proteins may then produce many physiological effects by acting as enzymes which control different metabolic reactions.

PITUITARY FUNCTIONS

The pituitary gland (hypophysis) is typically designated as "the master gland" and is divided into anterior and posterior lobes, adenohypophysis and neurohypophysis, respectively. However, one must not dismiss the importance of the hypothalamus, which actually controls the synthesis and the release of all products from this master gland.

141

The neurohypophysis is neurally attached to the hypothalamus and functions under the direct neural control of hypothalamic nuclei. The adenohypophysis is not attached neurally to the hypothalamus and is controlled via local hormones called "hypothalamic-releasing factors" which reach the cells of this pituitary region via a capillary system called the "hypothalamic-hypophyseal portal system." The hypothalamic-pituitary relationship is illustrated in Figure 13.1.

Figure 13.1 The hypothalamic-hypophyseal relationship.

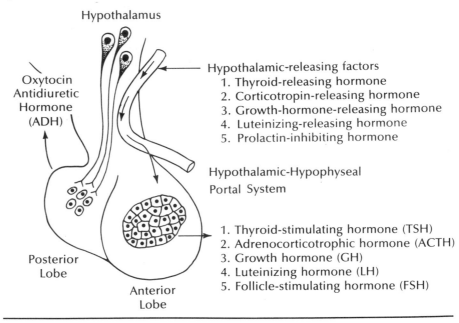

Hypothalamus

Oxytocin
Antidiuretic
Hormone
(ADH)

Hypothalamic-releasing factors
  1. Thyroid-releasing hormone
  2. Corticotropin-releasing hormone
  3. Growth-hormone-releasing hormone
  4. Luteinizing-releasing hormone
  5. Prolactin-inhibiting hormone

Hypothalamic-Hypophyseal
Portal System

  1. Thyroid-stimulating hormone (TSH)
  2. Adrenocorticotrophic hormone (ACTH)
  3. Growth hormone (GH)
  4. Luteinizing hormone (LH)
  5. Follicle-stimulating hormone (FSH)

Posterior
Lobe

Anterior
Lobe

Most of the hormones released by the pituitary gland stimulate other endocrine organs to synthesize and release their particular hormones. Therefore it is actually these latter organ products which are accountable for the beneficial metabolic effects. However, there are certain pituitary hormones which produce their own metabolic effects: somatotropin, oxytocin, and antidiuretic hormone (ADH).

Somatotropin (growth hormone) stimulates growth indirectly by causing the formation of somatomedin in the liver. This latter substance is actually the stimulus for cartilage and bone growth. However, growth hormone directly stimulates protein synthesis, fatty acid utilization, and decreased glucose utilization by cells.

The decreased cellular utilization of glucose may dramatically increase blood sugar levels, which serve to stimulate insulin release from the pancreas. This effect, combined with somatotropin's ability to directly stimulate insulin release by pancreatic beta cells may eventually produce "pancreas burnout" and subsequent diabetes mellitus. Until this occurs, the hyperglycemia induced by somatotropin produces a mild diabetic state called "pituitary diabetes."

Oxytocin stimulates the contraction of smooth muscle cells. This is most notable in the uterus and the myoepithelial cells of mammary glands. For these reasons, oxytocin is ascribed a critical role in childbirth and milk ejection.

Antidiuretic hormone (ADH) increases the permeability of collecting tubules in the kidney, which leads to water retention. It is also a very potent vasoconstrictor which accounts for its synonym, "vasopressin." Of particular interest is the inhibitory effect of alcohol on ADH release. Although this action occurs early following imbibition, circulating ADH levels continue to inhibit urination for 1 to 2 hours.

As stated previously, the remaining pituitary hormones act indirectly by promoting the synthesis and the release of hormones by other endocrine organs. The release of these "trophic" pituitary hormones is determined by the blood levels of the definitive hormone. For example, low blood levels of hydrocortisone (cortisol) are interpreted by the hypothalamus, which triggers the release of pituitary corticotropin (ACTH), which in turn stimulates the adrenal cortex to synthesize and release hydrocortisone. Conversely, high blood levels of hydrocortisone serve to inhibit further release of ACTH. This concept is often referred to as "negative feedback." Table 13.1 summarizes the pituitary hormones and their actions (see overleaf).

THYROID AND PARATHYROID FUNCTIONS

Thyroxine (T_4) and triiodothyronine (T_3) are the major products of the thyroid gland. Their synthesis and release into the bloodstream are controlled by TSH from the adenohypophysis. They stimulate metabolic functions in most body organs, and their lack results in a 40 to 50 percent reduction in the basal metabolic rate (BMR).

Thyroid follicles contain glycoprotein molecules called thyroglobulin. Each of these molecules contains 140 tyrosine molecules which are iodinated within the follicle. Thyroxin and triiodothyronine are formed from two tyrosine molecules which contain either three or four iodine atoms, T_3 and T_4. Under the influence of thyroid-stimulating hormone from the pituitary gland, protease enzymes cleave T_3 and T_4 units from the larger thyroglobulin molecule, and they diffuse into the blood stream. Thyroxine (T_4) comprises 90 percent of the normal thyroid hormone level, although T_3 is the more active hormone.

TABLE 13.1 Summary of pituitary hormones and their major actions

Hormone	Function
NEUROHYPOPHYSEAL	
oxytocin	uterine contraction, milk"let-down"
antidiuretic hormone (ADH)	water retention, vasoconstriction
ADENOHYPOPHYSEAL	
somatotropin (STH) (growth hormone)	stimulates cartilage and bone growth
adrenocorticotrophic hormone (ACTH, corticotropin)	stimulates hydrocortisone synthesis and release from adrenal cortex
luteinizing hormone (LH)	maintains corpus luteum
follicle-stimulating hormone (FSH)	stimulates ovum maturation
thyroid-stimulating hormone (TSH)	stimulates thyroxine synthesis and release from thyroid

The thyroid gland also synthesizes thyrocalcitonin, which functions to lower blood calcium levels. However, its action is very brief and not so critical in maintaining blood calcium levels as parathyroid hormone (parathormone).

Parathormone stimulates osteoclastic destruction of bone, thus liberating calcium into the blood stream. Its release is triggered by low calcium levels and is inhibited by high levels. The action of this hormone is very significant in regulating blood calcium levels, with thyrocalcitonin assuming a rather minor role.

PANCREATIC FUNCTIONS

Dispersed throughout the pancreas, between the digestive acini, are islands of cells called the "islets of Langerhans." Two of the three cellular types found in the islets are critical in regulating carbohydrate and fat metabolism. The beta cells release insulin which lowers blood sugar while glucagon, from the alpha cells, elevates blood sugar.

Insulin release is triggered by a sudden rise in blood sugar, such as that following a meal. By several mechanisms, insulin is able to lower the amount of free glucose found in blood. It promotes the storage of glucose within liver cells (glycogenesis), promotes the diffusion of glucose into most body cells (except brain tissue), and inhibits the formation of new glucose molecules (gluconeogenesis).

In addition to its effect on glucose metabolism, insulin inhibits lipolytic enzymes from hydrolizing triglycerides to free fatty acids. This effect of insulin is most evident in diabetic ketoacidosis where the lack of insulin permits large amounts of free fatty acids to be released. The oxidative metabolites of these acids, ketone bodies, produce the familiar "acetone breath" and metabolic acidosis.

Glucagon is released when blood sugar levels are low and functions to elevate blood sugar by freeing glucose from liver stores (glycogenolysis) and stimulating the formation of new glucose (gluconeogenesis). Glucagon is aided in its attempt to elevate blood sugar by two other hormones, hydrocortisone and epinephrine. Figure 13.2 illustrates the hormonal control of blood sugar levels.

Figure 13.2

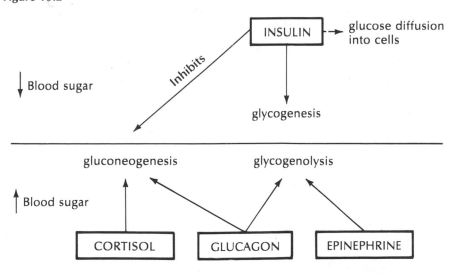

Blood sugar levels are lowered by promoting glucose storage (glycogenesis) and by inhibiting new glucose formation (gluconeogenesis). Blood sugar levels may be elevated by the stimulation of gluconeogenesis and glycogenolysis.

ADRENAL CORTEX FUNCTIONS

The adrenal cortex synthesizes two important classes of steroid hormones from cholesterol. The glucocorticoids, such as hydrocortisone (cortisol), are synthesized under the stimulus of ACTH and are concerned primarily with carbohydrate metabolism. The mineralocorticoids, such as aldosterone, are primarily controlled by the renin-angiotensin system and are concerned with sodium and water retention. A third class of steroid, the androgenic substances, are also formed in trace amounts but are physiologically insignificant unless hypercorticism occurs.

Glucocorticoids promote the formation of new glucose (gluconeogenesis) from amino acids mobilized from the protein of skeletal muscle, bone, and other tissues. They potentiate the lipolytic and cardiovascular effects of catecholamines, such as epinephrine. For these reasons, they are critical for the body to handle stressful situations. Their anti-inflammatory effects are not noticeable at normal physiological levels and will be discussed further in Chapter 15.

The mineralocorticoids are vital for fluid and electrolyte balance. This balance is critical for the proper function of most tissues but must be especially appreciated for its synergistic effect with glucocorticoids and catecholamines in cardiovascular function. Figure 13.3 illustrates the regulation of aldosterone and cortisol release from the adrenal cortex. The relationship between the hypothalamus, pituitary, and adrenal cortex in cortisol secretion is called the HPA axis.

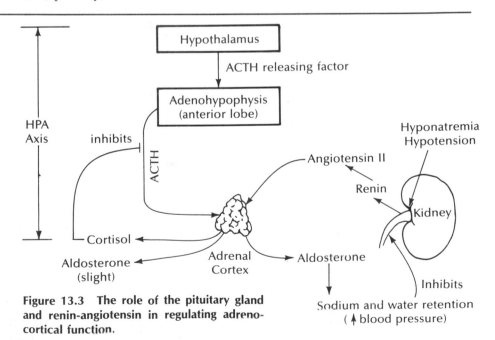

Figure 13.3 The role of the pituitary gland and renin-angiotensin in regulating adrenocortical function.

THE OVARIAN CYCLE

Under the influence of follicle-stimulating hormone (FSH) from the adenohypophysis, the primary follicles of the ovary begin to develop. After approximately 7 to 10 days, one follicle becomes prominent while the others regress. This one follicle and its egg will then continue to mature until the combination of FSH and luteinizing hormone (LH) causes ovulation to occur. LH will continue to maintain the remnant of the follicle (corpus luteum), which continues to produce estrogen and progesterone until blood levels reach a critical concentration. At this point, estrogen levels inhibit further FSH release, and later the progesterone inhibits LH release. With the loss of LH comes atrophy of the corpus luteum resulting in a loss of estrogen and progesterone secretion. In the absence of progesterone and estrogen, the endometrium sloughs, that is, the menses occur; and FSH is no longer inhibited resulting in a new cycle of follicular and egg development (see Figure 13.4). The major functions of estrogen are to mature and maintain all female sexual organs, (vagina, uterus, fallopian tubes, and breasts). Progesterone is often called the "hormone of pregnancy" because it functions to "ripen" and prepare the endometrium and secretory apparatus of the breasts for pregnancy and lactation.

Figure 13.4   The ovarian-pituitary relationship.

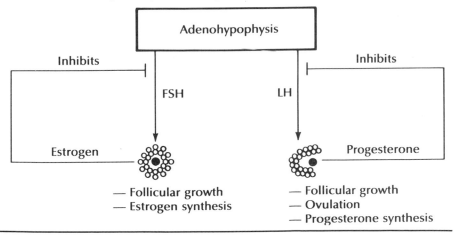

SUMMARY

The content of this chapter represents a cursory review of a very complex system. It is offered with the sole intention of providing the fundamentals with which you may grasp the therapeutic rationales discussed in the following chapter. A more detailed explanation may be obtained by consulting any physiology text.

14

Hormones and Antagonists

Most of the hormones discussed in the previous chapter either have been synthesized or extracted from animal tissue and are available as replacement therapy for hypofunctional states. It may also be possible in some cases to counteract hormonal actions in cases of hyperfunction. The logic of drug therapy discussed in this chapter builds on an understanding of normal endocrine function. Without mastery of the previous chapter, the contents of this chapter will prove difficult to understand.

THYROID DYSFUNCTION

Considering the positive action of thyroxine on so many body tissues, it is not surprising that symptoms of hypothyroidism, as well as hyperthyroidism, are numerous. Indeed myxedema and cretinism (hypothyroidism) may be viewed as a hypofunction of virtually every body organ system. While symptoms of hyperthyroidism may be equally ubiquitous, cardiovascular stimulation is the most notable cause for concern.

The therapy for various degrees of hypothyroidism generally involves replacement with thyroxine (Synthroid). The most notable side effects are cardiac in nature and consist of tachycardia, palpitations, and dysrhythmias. These effects may be counteracted with beta-adrenergic blockers, such as propranolol (Inderal), until a reduction in thyroxine concentration is accomplished.

There are three ways in which hyperthyroidism may be treated:

1. Inhibition of thyroxine synthesis.
2. Destruction of thyroid tissue by administering radioactive iodine.
3. Thyroidectomy.

The latter two methods are generally chosen following failure with the inhibiting agent, propylthiouracil (PTU). This drug competes for enzymes that iodinate the thyroglobulin precursor in the thyroid follicles. Side effects from this form of therapy are low, with agranulocytosis presenting the greatest source of concern.

ADRENOCORTICOSTEROIDS

In primary adrenal insufficiency states, such as Addison's disease, replacement therapy must include both aldosterone and hydrocortisone. If the condition is secondary to anterior pituitary insufficiency, ACTH (Acthar) replacement may stimulate adrenocortical function, thus eliminating the need for these agents. The most common use of adrenal steroids is in the treatment of inflammatory disorders and will be presented in the following chapter.

PANCREATIC HORMONES

Based on the underlying pathogenesis, several types of diabetes mellitus are described. However, the fundamental problem is either a relative or absolute insulin deficiency, which provides the basis for two major classes of diabetic patients. Those patients who require insulin replacement are called insulin-dependent (IDDM), and those who do not are called noninsulin-dependent (NIDDM).

Chronic complications of diabetes mellitus result from high blood glucose concentrations, which lead to abnormal glycoprotein formation with subsequent vascular compromise. The resulting ischemia then accounts for several "opathies," such as neuro-, nephro-, and retino-, as well as gangrenous limbs. The acute complications of hypoinsulinism result from insulin's normal inhibition of triglyceride catabolism. The ensuing ketoacidosis is the major finding in "diabetic coma."

> Noninsulin-dependent diabetics generally produce enough insulin to inhibit triglyceride catabolism, and therefore seldom suffer ketoacidotic episodes. In this regard, obese patients place such a demand on the "fat-sparing" function of insulin that inadequate amounts are available for glucose regulation. It may become necessary to place these patients on insulin replacement even though they do not suffer from absolute insulin lack.

In order to avoid these acute and chronic complications, the insulin-dependent diabetic must receive insulin replacement on a daily basis. Insulin, a polypeptide, is digested by the proteolytic enzymes, pepsin and trypsin, and for this reason cannot be administered orally. Although several parenteral concentrations are available (40, 100, and 500 units/ml), U-100 is the favored concentration and is encouraged as a standard concentration to avoid patient-dosing errors. The various preparations available differ in the speed of onset and the duration of action (see Table 14.1).

TABLE 14.1   Comparative onset and duration of action of commonly employed insulin preparations

Preparations	Onset (hrs.)	Duration (hrs.)
Fast-Acting		
insulin (regular)	.5–1	5–7
semilente insulin	1–3	12–16
Intermediate-Acting		
NPH insulin	2	24–28
lente insulin	2–4	24–28
Long-Acting		
ultralente insulin	4–6	36

The major side effect of insulin, hypoglycemia, is actually an exaggerated primary effect. Often referred to as "insulin shock," this condition is immediately threatening to CNS function since brain tissue is dependent on a continuous supply of serum glucose for energy. It is for this reason that any peculiar behavior in a diabetic patient should be treated with glucose replacement. Should the condition prove to be "hyperglycemic" in nature, the additional glucose will not worsen the condition since the major problem in "diabetic coma" generally relates to ketoacidosis, not the blood glucose levels.

Many diabetic patients are not truly insulin-dependent. These patients may be viewed as having "lazy pancreas," which can be stimulated by agents referred to as "oral hypoglycemics." These agents were discovered quite fortuitously in the 1940s by scientists researching the sulfonamide antimicrobial agents (sulfa drugs). Some of these agents were found to produce hypoglycemia as a side effect, and subsequently, were developed into the present group of oral hypoglycemic agents known as sulfonylureas (see Table 14.2). These agents all stimulate the pancreatic beta cells to produce insulin and, therefore, are useless in those patients with functionless islet cells, that is, IDDM. Drug interactions, cardiovascular side effects, and questionable long-term efficacy have placed this group of drugs in considerable controversy among many physicians.[1] The contemporary tendency is to manage noninsulin-dependent forms of diabetes with controlled diet and/or small daily doses of insulin.[2]

Glucagon is secreted by the alpha cells of the pancreas and produces actions opposite to those of insulin. Its major mechanism in raising blood sugar levels is by virtue of stimulating glycogenolysis in the liver. Its major use is in treating the hypoglycemia induced by insulin or the hypoglycemic agents. However, intravenous glucose administration is preferred initially since glucagon's action may be delayed (15 to 20 minutes) and may even prove futile should glycogen stores be depleted, which is typical in starvation states.

TABLE 14.2 Sulfonylurea oral hypoglycemics

tolbutamide (Orinase)	chlorpropamide (Diabinese)	glyburide (Micronase)
acetohexamide (Dymelor)	tolazamide (Tolinase)	glipizide (Glucuron, DiaBeta)

FEMALE SEX HORMONES

The terms estrogen and progestin are generic for the many natural and synthetic derivatives of estradiol and progesterone. Commercial preparations maintain all the actions of the natural hormones but resist their rapid hepatic biotransformation, making enteral administration quite acceptable. The normal metabolic functions of these hormones were presented in Chapter 13, and their use in replacement therapy is predicated on producing some or all of these effects.

The most frequent use of estrogen and progestin products is for their contraceptive action. The most popular oral contraceptives are referred to as "combination products" since each tablet contains an estrogen and a progestin. The estrogenic component inhibits FSH release, while the progestin inhibits LH and alters endometrial development. In the absence of these pituitary hormones, follicular development and ovulation are inhibited in virtually 100 percent of patients taking combination-type oral contraceptives. Contraception may also be accomplished by estrogens or progestins alone, for example, the "minipill," but side effects and menstrual irregularity make these preparations less desirable.

When used separately, estrogens and progestins are not so predictable in inhibiting FSH and LH release, and hence, ovulation. Therefore, local actions on the reproductive tract must be considered paramount. Chronic doses of progestins render the endometrium less functional for nidation of the blastocyst and also induce thicker mucus secretion in the cervix which opposes sperm motility.

High doses of estrogen administered post-coitally stimulate motility in the oviduct transporting the fertilized egg to the uterus before it has matured enough for nidation. Withdrawal from these large doses usually induces bleeding which obviously contributes to the abortafacient process.[3]

The most frequent side effects are attributed to estrogens and include nausea, thromboembolic disorders, and tumor growth. While these latter complications present a contraindication for estrogen use in those having a predisposition toward these diseases, the risks associated with pregnancy and childbirth are far greater. Table 14.3 lists the more popular preparations.

TABLE 14.3   Estrogen and progestin products

Estrogen Preparations
   diethylstilbestrol (Stilophostrol)
   estradiol (Progynon)
   conjugated estrogens (Premarin)

Progestin Preparations
   medroxyprogesterone (Provera)
   norethindrone (Micronor)

Combination Oral Contraceptives
   norethindrone and mestranol (Ortho-Novum)
   norgestrel and ethinyl estradiol (Ovral)
   Norinyl (same as Ortho-Novum)

Clomiphene (Clomid) is an anti-estrogenic agent which functions as an estrogen-receptor antagonist. The blockade of hypothalamic and pituitary receptors prevents the "negative-feedback" of estrogen on FSH release. The subsequent increase in FSH release heightens follicular growth and ovulation, rendering clomiphene quite useful for improving female fertility. As would be anticipated, the incidence of multiple births and ovarian follicular cyst formation are increased on taking this drug.

Some forms of breast cancer are estrogen-dependent as evidenced by the laboratory identification of estrogen receptors in biopsied tissue. The antagonistic action of clomiphene on this tissue has produced optimistic results in selected cases. This topic will be discussed further in Chapter 17.

SYNOPSIS OF THERAPEUTIC AGENTS

I. Thyroid hormone

   A. ACTION
      1. Stimulates many metabolic reactions
   B. USEFUL EFFECTS
      1. Corrects hypothyroid function
   C. PREPARATIONS
      1. Thyroxine (Synthroid)
   D. SECONDARY EFFECTS
      1. Tachycardia and palpitations

II. Insulin

   A. ACTION
      1. Stimulates glycogenesis and facilitates diffusion of glucose into cells

II. Insulin *(continued)*

B. USEFUL EFFECTS
   1. Lowers blood sugar
   2. Prevents catabolism of triglycerides
C. PREPARATIONS
   1. Insulin
   2. Diabinese
      a) Not actually insulin but stimulates insulin release from the pancreas
D. SECONDARY EFFECTS
   1. Hypoglycemia (insulin shock)

III. Glucagon

A. ACTION
   1. Stimulates glycogenolysis
B. USEFUL EFFECTS
   1. Raises blood sugar
C. SECONDARY EFFECTS
   1. Hyperglycemia

IV. Estrogen

A. Matures female sexual organs and inhibits FSH release
B. USEFUL EFFECTS
   1. Replacement therapy
   2. Contraception
   3. Decreased menopausal symptoms
C. PREPARATIONS
   1. Premarin
   2. Various birth control preparations
D. SECONDARY EFFECTS
   1. Thromboembolism
   2. Nausea
   3. Sodium and water retention

V. Progestins

A. ACTION
   1. Matures endometrium and breast tissue, and inhibits LH release

SYNOPSIS OF THERAPEUTIC AGENTS (*continued*)

V. Progestins *(continued)*

B. USEFUL EFFECTS
1. Regulates menstrual cycle
2. Maintains pregnancy
3. Contraception

C. PREPARATIONS
1. Provera
2. Micronor

D. SECONDARY EFFECTS
1. None significant

VI. Estrogen antagonists

A. ACTION
1. Block estrogen receptors permitting increased FSH release

B. USEFUL EFFECTS
1. Improves fertility

C. PREPARATIONS
1. Clomid

D. SECONDARY EFFECTS
1. Ovarian cyst formation

ARTICLES FOR DISCUSSION

1. **Fletcher, H. P.** 1976. The oral antidiabetic drugs: Pro and con. *American Journal of Nursing* 76:596.
2. **Shen, S. W., and Bressler, R.** 1977. Clinical pharmacology of oral antidiabetic agents. *New England Journal of Medicine* 296:787–793.
3. **Yve, D. K., and Turtle, J. R.** 1977. New forms of insulin and their use in the treatment of diabetes. *Diabetes* 26:341–347.
4. **Kolata, G. B.** 1979. Controversy over study of diabetes drugs continues for nearly a decade. *Science* 203:986–990.
5. **Galloway, J. A.** 1980. Insulin treatment for the early '80s: Facts and questions about old and new insulins and their usage. *Diabetes Care* 3:615–622.
6. **Waits, L. F.** 1983. Managing diabetics during surgery. *AORN Journal* 37:928–941.

7. **Dickerson, J.** 1983. The Pill: A closer look. *American Journal of Nursing* 83:1392–1398.

8. **Hulka, B. D., et al.** 1982. Protection against endometrial carcinoma by combination-product oral contraceptives. *JAMA* 247:475–477.

9. **Stadel, B. V.** 1981. Oral contraceptives and cardiovascular disease. *New England Journal of Medicine* 305:612–618, 672–677.

10. **Hallal, J.** 1977. Thyroid disorders. *American Journal of Nursing* 77:417–432.

REFERENCES

1. **Kolata, G. B.** Controversy over study of diabetes drugs continues for nearly a decade. *Science* 203: 986–990.

2. **Goodman, L. S., and Gilman, A.** 1980. *The Pharmacological Basis of Therapeutics.* 6th ed. New York: Macmillan, pp. 1513–1514.

3. Ibid. pp. 1441–1442

15

Anti-Inflammatory Drugs

Inflammation is a vascular and cellular response to injury. The process is remarkably similar regardless of the nature of injury. Indeed the cardinal signs of redness, heat, swelling, and pain are seen following injury from trauma, infection, or allergy. For this reason, the suffix "-itis" tells us only that the organ is inflamed, not the cause of the inflammation.

The inflammatory process may be viewed as three phases: vascular, fluid exudation, and cellular exudation. However, one must realize that, by the time signs are clinically evident, all phases are occurring simultaneously.

Following injury to tissues, chemicals are synthesized and/or released by the injured cells. These so-called "inflammatory mediators" dilate vessels and increase the permeability of their walls. As a result of vasodilation, there is increased blood flow, hyperemia, which provides the cardinal signs of redness and warmth. The increased permeability allows exudation of plasma and leukocytes into the injured region, which results in swelling and pain from the buildup of pressure.

From this description, the key role of the inflammatory mediators is quite obvious. The fundamental concept of anti-inflammatory drug action is the interference with the synthesis and/or the action of these mediators. The most studied inflammatory mediators are histamine, bradykinin, prostaglandins, and the leukotrienes, previously named the slow-reacting substance of anaphylaxis (SRS-A). Some of these mediators not only affect the blood vessels directly but facilitate the inflammatory activity of the various leukocytes.

The inflammatory process may be viewed as a "Dr. Jekyll–Mr. Hyde" phenomenon. While being absolutely vital in our protection from injury and infection, it may also become so exaggerated as to constitute a disease entity of its own. It is for this latter reason that anti-inflammatory drugs are so essential.

156

NONSTEROIDAL AGENTS

Following injury, arachidonic acid is released from cell membranes and is converted into chemicals called prostaglandins. The enzyme system that controls this reaction is appropriately termed prostaglandin synthetase. The nonsteroidal anti-inflammatory drugs (NSAIDS) inhibit these enzymes, thereby preventing the synthesis of these inflammatory mediators. In Chapter 11 we discussed the role of prostaglandins in producing pain and fever, pointing out that most of the nonnarcotic agents exert their analgesic and antipyretic effects by inhibiting their synthesis. Since these substances are also inflammatory mediators, their inhibition should result in a depression of the inflammatory process. It is by this mechanism that the NSAIDS exert their primary effect.

TABLE 15.1   Nonsteroidal anti-inflammatory drugs and typical daily dosage ranges

Preparations	Dose Range
aspirin	4000-6000 mg
ibuprofen (Motrin)	1600-2400 mg
naproxen (Naprosyn)	500- 750 mg
sulindac (Clinoril)	300- 400 mg
indomethacin (Indocin)	50- 200 mg
phenylbutazone (Butazolidin)	300- 600 mg
fenoprofen (Nalfon)	1200-2400 mg
tolmetin (Tolectin)	600-1800 mg
piroxicam (Feldene)	20 mg
meclofenamate (Meclomen)	200- 400 mg
diflunisal (Dolobid)	500-1000 mg

Aspirin is the prototype of the NSAIDS and was described in Chapter 11. While being quite effective in reducing inflammation, it is not very potent. You will recall that typical analgesic doses range from 300 to 1000 mgs, but anti-inflammatory efficacy is not attained with doses less than 4 to 6 grams on a daily basis. Many patients are able to tolerate this dosage and therefore take advantage of this inexpensive treatment for chronic inflammatory disorders. However, for those who cannot tolerate this amount of aspirin the more potent NSAIDS offer a more expensive alternative. Table 15.1 lists the popular NSAIDS with their daily anti-inflammatory dosages. While studies conflict on comparative anti-inflammatory efficacies, it is generally agreed that indomethacin and phenylbutazone are superior, but are associated with more serious side effects, including depressed hematopoietic function. Indeed phenylbutazone may produce aplastic anemia and agranulocytosis in a significant number of patients. For this reason it is recommended only for short-term use (one week). If the drug is used for longer periods, blood cell counts must be taken frequently.

The role of prostaglandins in producing pain and inflammation following surgery has prompted a number of studies employing NSAIDS preoperatively to reduce the intensity of postoperative pain and swelling.[1]

STEROIDAL AGENTS

The normal physiological roles of the adrenocorticosteroids were discussed in the preceding chapter. At higher than physiological doses, the glucocorticoids possess dramatic anti-inflammatory efficacy. Hydrocortisone possesses some mineralocorticoid activity (sodium and water retention), and is therefore not commonly used for long-term anti-inflammatory therapy. The synthetic derivatives are purer "glucocorticoids" and therefore are less likely to produce this undesirable effect.

Glucocorticoids inhibit all phases of the inflammatory process and thereby suppress all of the cardinal signs. This must not be taken lightly, since we rely on these signs for diagnostic purposes. It must be further emphasized that these agents do nothing to counteract the cause of the inflammation and, should it be infection, the patient will be both "signless" as well as "defenseless"!

> There are many mechanisms by which the glucocorticoids inhibit the inflammatory process. They directly depress lymphoid tissue, thereby inhibiting the cellular role of lymphocytes in chronic inflammation and graft rejection. They stabilize lysosomal membranes, preventing release of enzymes that continue to incite the inflammatory response. There is also substantial evidence that they inhibit the release of arachidonic acid, which serves as the precursor for prostaglandin synthesis.[2,3]

Table 15.2 lists the glucocorticoids employed in the therapy of inflammatory disease. Although differing in potency, none have been shown to be superior in efficacy; and for this reason, prednisone (the least expensive) is most popular for chronic use.

The complications from steroid therapy are numerous. One must consider that all normal actions of glucocorticoids are going to be pronounced, considering the high dose required to attain an anti-inflammatory effect. In fact it is convenient to describe all the effects collectively as "cushingoid symptoms" since we are actually inducing an "iatrogenic hypercorticism." Of course, if we are employing pure glucocorticoid agents, the sodium- and water-retaining symptoms of classic

Cushing's syndrome are not so obvious. The hyperglycemic action of glucocorticoids poses a particular problem in diabetic patients, and all patients must be cautioned concerning their lack of resistance to infection. Steroids are also known to aggravate peptic ulcer, elevate mood, and cause osteoporosis and myopathy.

> The exact mechanisms by which steroids produce these effects is not well-established. However, they do inhibit calcium absorption, and the resultant parathyroid activity accounts for bone decalcification and subsequent osteoporosis (steroid fractures). Added to this is evidence that corticosteroids inhibit osteoblastic function.[4]

In addition to the above side effects, chronic therapy maintains blood levels high enough to inhibit diurnal ACTH release from the adenohypophysis. By depressing this hypothalamic-pituitary-adrenal (HPA) axis, the adrenal cortex is not stimulated and undergoes a form of disuse atrophy. Should the patient experience severe stress, such as infection or surgery, ACTH release will not be able to awaken the atrophied adrenal cortex. Without these adrenocorticosteroids to raise blood sugar and potentiate catecholamines, the patient will go into a shocklike syndrome referred to as "adrenal crisis." To circumvent this possibility, it is typical to administer a "steroid-prep" to these patients before any surgical procedure. This usually consists of 100 to 200 mg of Solu-Cortef intravenously.

TABLE 15.2 Glucocorticosteroids and dosages equivalent to 20 mg of hydrocortisone (while potencies and mineralocorticoid activity vary, anti-inflammatory efficacy is comparable)

Agent	Dose	Mineralocorticoid Activity
hydrocortisone (Cortef et al.)	20 mg	Significant
prednisone (Deltasone et al.)	5 mg	Slight
prednisolone (Delta-Cortef et al.)	5 mg	Slight
methylprednisolone (Medrol et al.)	4 mg	Slight
triamcinolone (Kenalog et al.)	4 mg	Slight to none
betamethasone (Celestone)	.6 mg	None
dexamethasone (Decadron et al.)	.75 mg	None

Alternate day therapy (ADT) is designed to prevent adrenal atrophy from occurring in patients who must be maintained on chronic steroid therapy. On the alternating days a steroid is not taken, the HPA axis is functional and ACTH is able to stimulate cortical function, thus preventing the prolonged inactivity that results in atrophy. Unfortunately, some inflammatory diseases cannot be controlled with this method, and daily doses are a necessity. If a steroid is to be terminated, it must be done gradually over a prolonged period until adrenal function is able to recover. In fact, total recovery may not occur for 6 to 12 months after all steroid medication is withdrawn. For this reason "steroid preps" may still be indicated prior to surgery for those patients recently withdrawn from steroid therapy.

Glucocorticoids are employed for many reasons on an acute or short-term basis for allergic reactions, IV extravasations, and trauma. None of the side effects discussed are applicable in these situations. A few days of even large doses of glucocorticosteroids are virtually free of side effects except for mood elevation and resultant insomnia.

HISTAMINE BLOCKERS

Drugs which act as antagonists on histamine receptors may be referred to as histamine blockers, or more typically, antihistamines. They are not actually considered anti-inflammatory agents because of the limited role of histamine in chronic inflammatory conditions. Their major efficacy is seen in hypersensitivity reactions in which histamine produces urticaria (hives) and itching. They will not reverse the hypotension and the bronchospasm of anaphylactoid reactions which are produced by mediators other than histamine. In this situation, epinephrine is the "lifesaver," with subsequent administration of antihistamines and steroids serving only to reduce any itching or urticaria.

The most common side effect of antihistamines is sedation, which requires that patients be cautioned against overzealous consumption of other CNS depressants while taking antihistamine preparations. As stated in Chapter 9, several antihistamines, for example, Vistaril, are employed intentionally as sedative agents.

Most antihistamines possess antiemetic efficacy and may be employed to counteract nausea and vomiting. This is especially true when employing them concurrently with narcotic analgesics. Diphenhydramine (Benadryl) is generally considered the prototype of this drug class.

In addition to its inflammatory role, histamine stimulates hydrochloric acid release in the stomach. In this location, however, the histamine receptor (H_2) is different from those mediating urticaria and itching (H_1). Cimetidine (Tagamet) and ranitidine (Zantac) are specific H_2 receptor blockers. They lack any significant sedative or antiemetic actions attributed to the H_1 blockers and are used solely for their inhibitory action on gastric acid release. Their discovery has led to impressive results in the therapy of peptic ulcer.

The identification of two histamine receptor subtypes, H_1 and H_2 further explains the inability of the H_1 blockers (Benadryl) to reverse the vasodilation and hypotension associated with anaphylactoid reactions and narcotic administration. It appears that histamine dilates blood vessels by stimulating both H_1 and H_2 receptors on vascular smooth muscle. Blocking only H_1 receptors is insufficient to reverse this effect.[5]

SYNOPSIS OF THERAPEUTIC AGENTS

I. NSAIDS

A. ACTION
1. Inhibit synthesis of prostaglandins
B. USEFUL EFFECTS
1. Anti-inflammatory
2. Analgesia
3. Antipyretic
C. PREPARATIONS
1. Aspirin
2. Naprosyn
3. Indocin
D. SECONDARY EFFECTS
1. GI disturbances
a) Bleeding
b) Irritation
c) Nausea
2. Inhibit platelet aggregation

II. Glucocorticosteroids

A. ACTION
1. Depress all aspects of inflammation
B. USEFUL EFFECTS
1. Anti-inflammatory
C. PREPARATIONS
1. Hydrocortisone (Solu-Cortef)
2. Prednisone
3. Dexamethasone (Decadron)

SYNOPSIS OF THERAPEUTIC AGENTS (*continued*)

II. Glucocorticosteroids *(continued)*

    D. SECONDARY EFFECTS

        1. Hyperglycemia

        2. CNS Stimulation

        3. Osteoporosis

        4. Decreased resistance to infection

        5. Adrenal Atrophy

III. **Antihistamines**

    A. ACTION

        1. Block histamine receptors

    B. USEFUL EFFECTS

        1. Counteract itching and hives

        2. Sedation

        3. Antiemetic

    C. PREPARATIONS

        1. Diphenhydramine (Benadryl)

        2. Chlorpheniramine (Chlor-Trimeton)

        3. Cimetidine (Tagamet)

            a) Blocks only gastric acid secretion

    D. SECONDARY EFFECTS

        1. Sedation

        2. Dry mouth

ARTICLES FOR DISCUSSION

1. **Simon, L. J., and Mills, J. A.** 1980. Nonsteroidal anti-inflammatory drugs. *New England Journal of Medicine* 302:1179–1185, 1237–1242.
2. **Tatro, D. S., et al.** 1980. Nonsteroidal anti-inflammatory agents' effects on platelet function. *Hospital Formulary* 15:932–935.
3. **Toogood, J. H.** 1982. How to use steroids in asthma therapy. *Journal of Respiratory Diseases* 3:15–22.
4. **McDonough, A. L.** 1982. Effects of corticosteroids on Articular cartilage: A review of the literature. *Physical Therapy* 55:835–839.
5. **Kleinkort, J. A., and Wood F.** 1975. Phonophoresis with one percent versus 10 percent hydrocortisone. *Physical Therapy* 55:1320–1324.
6. **Baylink, D. J.** 1983. Glucocorticoid-induced osteoporosis. *New England Journal of Medicine* 309:306–308.
7. **Bahn, S. L.** 1982. Glucocorticosteroids in dentistry. *Journal of the American Dental Association* 105:476–487.
8. **Manchi, L., et al.** 1982. Cimetidine and related drugs in anesthesia. *Anesthesia and Analgesia* 61:595–605.
9. **West, et al.** 1975. A review of antihistamines and the common cold. *Pediatrics* 56:100–107.
10. **Jensen, R. T., et al.** 1983. Cimetidine-induced impotence and breast changes in patients with gastric hypersecretory states. *New England Journal of Medicine* 308:883–887.

REFERENCES

1. **Dionne, R. A., and Cooper S. A.** 1978. Evaluation of preoperative ibuprofen for postoperative pain after removal of third molars. *Oral Surgery* 45:851.
2. **Hong, S. L., and Levine L. S.** 1976. Inhibition of arachidonic acid release from cells as the biochemical action of anti-inflammatory corticosteroids. *Proceedings of the National Academy of Sciences of the USA* 73:1730–1734.
3. **Claman, H. N.** 1975. How corticosteroids work. *Journal of Allergy and Clinical Immunology* 55:145–151.
4. **Hahn, T. J.** 1978. Corticosteroid-induced osteopenia. *Archives of Internal Medicine* 138:882–885.
5. **Philbin, D. M.** 1981. The use of H_1 and H_2 histamine antagonists with morphine anesthesia: A double-blind study. *Anesthesiology* 55:292.

16

Antimicrobial Agents

As the name implies, antimicrobial agents are drugs used to combat infection. They include antibacterial, antifungal, antiviral, and many other subclasses of agents. The term "antibiotic" is strictly reserved for those agents derived from living microorganisms, but this definition is no longer useful considering the number of semi-synthetic and synthetic agents introduced each year. For this reason, it is generally acceptable to use the terms "antibacterial" and "antibiotic" interchangeably.

Fundamental to antimicrobial action is the concept of selective toxicity. This is to say that these agents must inhibit or destroy microbial cells without damaging human cells. Structural and metabolic differences between microbial and human cells have been identified and form the basis for the selective action of most antimicrobial agents. The bacterial cell wall represents the most striking difference and presents a very selective site of action for antimicrobial drugs. The penicillins and the cephalosporins are remarkably effective agents and produce few side effects because of their specific site of action on cell-wall synthesis. Microbial cell membranes, ribosomes, and certain metabolic pathways also differ from human cells and offer the principal remaining sites of action. Table 16.1 categorizes the four major sites of antimicrobial action.

TABLE 16.1   Major mechanisms and sites of action of antimicrobial drugs

1. Alter cell-membrane permeability **a)** nystatin **b)** amphotericin B	**3.** Inhibit protein synthesis at various ribosomal units **a)** aminoglycosides **c)** erythromycins **b)** tetracyclines
2. Inhibit cell-wall synthesis **a)** penicillins **b)** cephalosporins	**4.** Alter purine synthesis **a)** sulfonamides **b)** trimethoprim

---

Antimicrobial agents may be utilized to treat infection or to prevent infection from occurring. There is no dispute regarding the presurgical use of antimicrobial drugs to prevent either bacterial endocarditis or infection of certain orthopedic protheses. However, the routine surgical use of antimicrobial prophylaxis is heavily debated, and its practice continues to vary among surgeons.

Patients with organic (structural) cardiac defects are at risk of developing bacterial endocarditis following any surgical procedure. For this reason, the American Heart Association has presented guidelines for antimicrobial prophylaxis in these patients.[1]

Routine indiscriminate prophylactic use of these agents in all surgical patients is debatable. However, it is considered acceptable to choose agents specific for pathogens most likely to infect the specific surgical region. The drug should be administered less than 4 hours preoperatively and should not continue for more than a 24-hour period.[2, 3]

Before discussing the individual classes, issues common to all antimicrobial agents should be addressed. Since most agents are selective for specific groups of microbes, unaffected organisms may overgrow and produce "superinfections." A common example is when *Candida* infection follows antibacterial therapy. Since bacteria normally depress fungal growth, inhibiting this former group permits fungi to reproduce rapidly, resulting in a fungal superinfection.

When taken orally, most antimicrobial agents alter intestinal microflora to a point that diarrhea and GI upset may occur. In some cases a category of "superinfection" may occur in which the overgrown species produces toxins that precipitate ulcerations of the intestinal tract. This is the mechanism by which clindamycin (Cleocin) produces a pseudomembranous colitis.

The appearance of resistant microbial strains is a universal concern, and the indiscriminate use of antimicrobial agents is contributing to this problem. There are many mechanisms by which antimicrobial resistance develops, but selective inhibition must be considered a major mechanism. While penicillin is bacteriocidal to most gram-positive cocci, there are always mutants, for example, *Staphylococcus aureus,* which are resistant. During a 7 to 10 day course of penicillin therapy, mutant species may reproduce at will and reside not only in the patient but in the immediate environment. It is because of the concentrated use of antimicrobial agents in hospitals, that these institutions harbor some of our most resistant organisms, such as *S. aureus* and *Pseudomonas aeruginosa.* It is these microorganisms that are most significant in producing nosocomial infections in hospitalized patients.

SULFONAMIDES

The sulfonamides (sulfa drugs) were the first antimicrobial agents introduced for treating bacterial infection. Until penicillins and other antibiotics were available, frequent sulfonamide use led to the development of resistant microbial strains, which continue to limit the spectrum of this class. However, sulfonamides continue to be effective in the treatment of urinary-tract infections.

The sulfonamides extent their bacteriostatic effect by a classic antimetabolite mechanism. They closely resemble para-aminobenzoic acid (PABA) in structure and compete with it during the synthesis of folic acid (Figure 16.1). Obviously, microbes which do not synthesize their own folic acid are insensitive to this class of agent. Human cells are exemplary of this latter category since our source of folic acid is dietary.

The sulfonamides are capable of a wide range of adverse effects, but various types of hypersensitivity reactions are most frequent. Renal toxicity from crystal formation and various blood dyscrasias are possible but are infrequent with sulfisoxazole (Gantrisin) and other more soluble agents.

The combination of sulfamethoxazole and trimethoprim (Bactrim, Septra) has established itself as a very effective regimen against organisms resistant to

Figure 16.1
Trimethoprim and sulfonamides produce a synergistic antimicrobial action by inhibiting two steps in purine synthesis. Microorganisms resistant to sulfa drug action may still be unable to reduce the folic acid to tetrahydrofolate by virtue of trimethoprim's action.

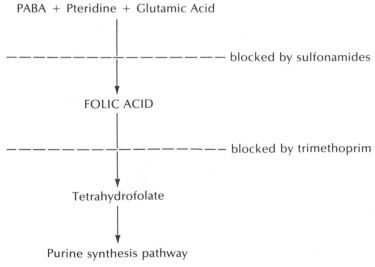

PABA + Pteridine + Glutamic Acid

—————————————————— blocked by sulfonamides

FOLIC ACID

—————————————————— blocked by trimethoprim

Tetrahydrofolate

Purine synthesis pathway

sulfonamides alone. Figure 16.1 illustrates the synergistic action of sulfonamides and trimethoprim in inhibiting the folic acid pathway.

The sulfonamide preparations are most commonly employed for urinary-tract infections and otitis media. However, topical preparations are also available for use during bowel surgery; and there are recurrent pulmonary and sinus infections that may respond to the combination of sulfamethoxazole and trimethoprim.

PENICILLINS

What is generally referred to as "the golden age of antimicrobial therapy" began in 1941 with the production of penicillin for patient use.

> The first trial of penicillin in the United States occurred in 1942 at New Haven Hospital, Yale University. The patient was a 33-year old female suffering infection following abortion of a four-month fetus. Sulfonamides were ineffective and the patient continued a critical downhill course. The supply of penicillin was so limited that it was recovered from her urine for reuse during the first week of therapy. A purer supply became available for two more weeks of therapy, following which, the patient dramatically recovered.[4]

The penicillins exert their bacteriocidal effect by inhibiting cell-wall synthesis. The prototype, penicillin G, has a fairly limited spectrum of activity, that is, gram-positive cocci, *Neisseria gonorrhea*, *Treponema pallidum*. However, given the frequency of infections caused by these particular microorganisms, penicillins are still among the most widely used antimicrobial agents. Although available for enteral administration, penicillin G is unpredictably absorbed from the GI tract and is therefore generally administered parenterally. Penicillin V is better absorbed and is the preferred form for oral administration.

> Penicillin is acidic and is combined with several bases to form salts for parenteral administration. The salts differ in rate of absorption from muscle depots. Potassium salts may be administered IM, but their primary route is IV. Procaine and benzathine salts are designed for IM administration and must *never* be injected intravenously. Figure 16.2 illustrates the rate of absorption and the duration of blood titer following IM injection of the three salt preparations. By studying this graph, the advantages of the various salt preparations will be apparent.

Many penicillin derivatives are available which offer advantages over penicillin G and V. Ampicillin is the prototype of those agents possessing a broader

Figure 16.2 Penicillin plasma concentrations following IM administration of various parenteral forms.

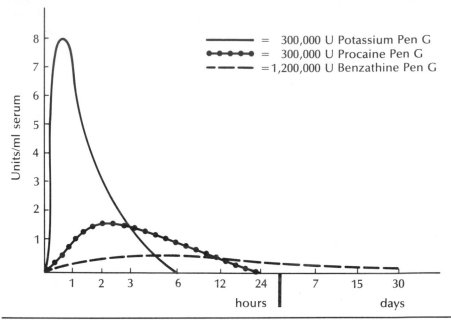

spectrum of activity including many gram-negative organisms. Many species of microbes are resistant to penicillins because of their ability to synthesize penicillinase, an enzyme which destroys penicillin. The prototype of the penicillins which resist this enzymatic destruction is methicillin and is indicated for the treatment of *S. aureus* infections which are the most notable penicillinase producers. Since many methicillin-resistant strains have been identified, other members of this penicillin class are usually preferred (see Table 16.2).

Figure 16.3 illustrates the portion of the penicillin molecule cleaved by penicillinase. This beta lactam ring is also found in cephalosporin agents and may be destroyed by cephalosporinases. Many types of bacterial enzymes are able to destroy penicillin and/or cephalosporin and are logically referred to collectively as the beta lactamases.

The penicillins are the least toxic of all antimicrobial agents and therefore may be administered in heroic doses without adverse consequences. Their major shortcoming is allergenicity with incidence reports ranging anywhere from 1 to 10

TABLE 16.2 Commonly Employed Penicillin Preparations and their Major Spectrum of Activity

Preparation	*Spectrum*
penicillin G, V	Streptococci, *Neisseria*, spirochetes
ampicillin amoxacillin	all above plus *E. coli* and other gram-negative microbes
methicillin oxacillin nafcillin	*Staphylococcus aureus* plus penicillin G spectrum
carbenicillin ticarcillin piperacillin azlocillin mezlocillin	extended spectrum to include many *Pseudomonas* species

Figure 16.3 Comparative structure of penicillins and cephalosporins.

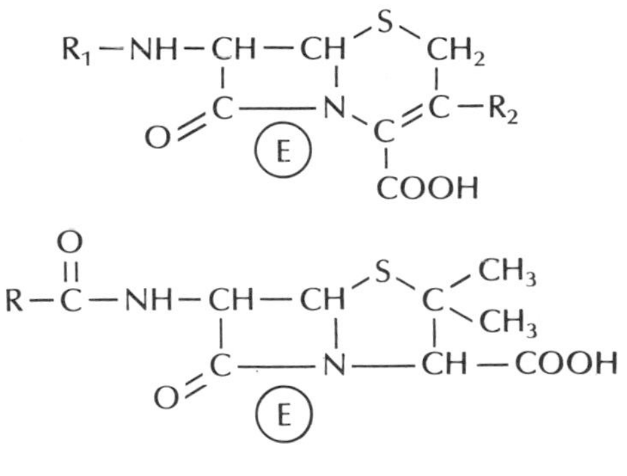

Cephalosporins

Penicillins

Ⓔ is the site of beta lactamase activity, that is, penicillinase and cephalosporinase.

percent of the patient population. Many of the skin reactions may not be truly allergic in nature, but the consequences of a major anaphylactic reaction hardly justifies challenging the issue. It has been estimated that 300 deaths each year may be attributed to penicillin anaphylaxis. This may not necessarily implicate penicillin as more antigenic than other antibiotics since it may also be indicative of penicillin's frequent use. The commonly used penicillins are listed in Table 16.2.

CEPHALOSPORINS

These agents are similar in structure and action to the penicillins with the two groups often referred to as the "beta lactam antibiotics." More than any other antibiotic class, the cephalosporins are exerting the greatest impact on hospital formulary costs. The intense marketing strategies of manufacturers have promoted the use of these expensive agents when other, less expensive agents may be equally efficacious. This is not to say that certain cephalosporin derivatives do not offer advantages in special circumstances—only that many gram-positive infections may be treated at considerably less expense with the penicillins. New cephalosporins are being introduced continuously and they are grouped according to "generations," that is, first, second, and third generation cephalosporins. Table 16.3 lists examples of each generation, their approximate daily cost, and their general spectrum of activity.

Cephalosporins produce a low incidence of nephrotoxicity, most notably in renal-compromised patients and when combined with other nephrotoxic agents. However, the major adverse effect of these agents is hypersensitivity, which is hardly remarkable considering their structural similarity to the penicillins. Continuing this line of reasoning, one would suspect a potential for cross-hypersensitivity in patients allergic to penicillin. While documented, this occurrence is not sufficiently frequent to contraindicate cephalosporins in patients with histories of only mild reactions to penicillins. However, a past history of a major penicillin reaction must be considered an absolute contraindication for cephalosporin use.[5]

TABLE 16.3   General Antimicrobial Spectrum and Daily Cost for Parental Administration of Cephalosporins Compared to Ampicillin

Preparation	Cost*	Spectrum
ampicillin	$ 88	Streptococci, *H. influenza,* many gram-negative microbes
cephalothin (Keflin) (first generation)	92	similar spectrum to ampicillin with addition of *Klebsiella* species
cefamandole (Mandol) (second generation)	103	more gram-negatives than above and specifically enterobacteria species resistant to many beta lactamases
cefotaxine (Claforan) (third generation)	162	very broad spectrum, including some gram-negative rods and resistant to many beta lactamases

*Approximate daily cost in dollars to the hospitalized patient. It is obvious that cost differences may become quite significant during a 7- to 14-day course of therapy.

ERYTHROMYCINS

Erythromycins may exert either a bacteriostatic or bacteriocidal effect, depending on the organism and the concentration of the drug. It exerts its effect by binding to bacterial ribosomes, thereby interfering with protein synthesis. Since it produces a high incidence of nausea, doses administered orally are generally not large enough to produce bacteriocidal levels and, as is the case with all bacteriostatic agents, the patient's immune system is ultimately responsible for clearing the infection.

Erythromycin's spectrum is fairly similar to that of penicillin, and therefore receives its major use as an alternative in patients allergic to penicillin. Legionnaires' disease is one of a very limited number of infections for which erythromycin is considered the primary agent of choice. Table 16.4 lists common erythromycin preparations.

TABLE 16.4 Erythromycin Preparations Including Various Salts Designed to Resist Gastric Acid Degradation (providing greater availability for absorption in the small intestine)

Generic Name	Brand Name
Erythromycin base	(E-mycin* et al.)
Erythromycin stearate	(Erythrocin et al.)
Erythromycin ethylsuccinate	(E.E.S. et al.)
Erythromycin estolate	(Ilosone)

*enteric-coated

TETRACYCLINES

Tetracyclines exert their bacteriostatic effect by inhibiting protein synthesis at bacterial ribosomes. They possess the broadest spectrum of activity among antimicrobial agents. While they may be used for a variety of infections, their greatest use is in the treatment of acne, sinusitis, and respiratory-tract infections.

The tetracyclines chelate to bivalent cations, such as calcium, which creates several clinically significant problems. Consumption with dairy products and antacids hinders absorption, which is not impressive even under ideal conditions. They tend to store in calcified tissues, which may result in poor bone formation and staining of tooth enamel in infants and children. This latter effect is significant only when enamel is forming since mature enamel does not exhibit the calcium dynamics of osseous tissue. It is generally considered prudent to avoid this drug in the pregnant mother and in children up to seven years of age to avoid "tetracycline staining." This restriction is not significant considering the number of alternative agents available.

Some of the tetracyclines may produce a skin reaction in sunlight called phototoxicity. This requires that patients be warned to avoid sunbathing while taking this medication. Both liver and kidney toxicity are possible but not frequent with typical doses. Doxycycline (Vibramycin) is excreted totally in the feces and is the obvious choice in patients with compromised renal function. This preparation is absorbed better than other tetracyclines and can be administered once daily which is a considerable advantage over t.i.d. (three times daily) and q.i.d. (four times daily) regimens in terms of patient compliance. Table 16.5 lists the tetracycline preparations and their half-lives. Since their antibacterial spectrum is broad, *Candida* superinfections are not uncommon when using any of these preparations.

TABLE 16.5   Tetracyclines

Preparation	Half-Life (hrs.)
Short*	
Tetracycline (Achromycin, et al.)	8
Oxytetracycline (Terramycin)	9
Intermediate*	
Demeclocycline (Declomycin)	12
Methacycline (Rondomycin)	14
Long*	
Minocycline (Minocin)	16
Doxycycline (Vibramycin)	18

*Tetracyclines may be classified as short-, intermediate-, and long-acting based on their half-life.

Although it is not a tetracycline, chloramphenicol (Chloromycetin) is very similar to this class in spectrum and action. Its greater efficacy is offset by its significant incidence of bone marrow toxicity resulting in pancytopenia, of which aplastic anemia is most significant. It is quite valuable in combination with one or two other agents in the "shotgun" treatment of life-threatening infections in which the primary pathogens have not yet been identified. When more specific agents can be selected, the chloramphenicol is discontinued since it is considered the agent of choice only in salmonella typhi infections.

AMINOGLYCOSIDES

These agents are bacteriocidal primarily against gram-negative bacilli, which are the primary pathogens in many life-threatening infections involving virtually any organ system. No other antimicrobial class can claim comparable efficacy against these organisms. Unfortunately their renal and cranial nerve VIII toxicity (ototoxicity) requires careful patient monitoring when employing any aminoglycoside derivative. This neurotoxicity may involve auditory and vestibular components and thereby impair hearing and/or balance.

> To avoid nephrotoxicity with these agents, it is common to monitor serum creatinine and aminoglycoside blood levels during therapy. "Trough" levels are taken just prior to administration of the next dose, and "peak" levels are taken one hour after the dose is administered. Trough levels must be higher than 2 mcg/ml to maintain antimicrobial activity while peak levels greater than 10 mcg/ml are more frequently associated with nephrotoxicity.[6, 7]

Gentamicin (Garamycin) and tobramycin (Nebcin) are the most frequently employed aminoglycosides. Tobramycin appears to be less nephrotoxic and is slightly more active against *Pseudomonas aeruginosa*.[6, 7] If these are not primary considerations, gentamicin is preferred based on its comparable efficacy and lesser cost.

Streptomycin is still used in severe cases of tuberculosis but has been largely replaced by the combination of isoniazid and rifampin. Streptomycin is still utilized along with other agents in the treatment and prophylaxis of bacterial endocarditis in those patients with valvular replacements.

Amikacin (Amikin) is a semi-synthetic preparation which is not destroyed by most of the inactivating enzymes produced by microorganisms resistant to other aminoglycosides. Since most other characteristics are similar to those of gentamicin, many infectious disease experts believe amikacin's primary use should be restricted to the treatment of those infections caused by gentamicin and tobramycin-resistant organisms. Table 16.6 lists aminoglycoside preparations and compares their relative nephrotoxicity and ototoxicity. (See next page.)

ANTIFUNGAL AGENTS

Nystatin (Mycostatin) and amphotericin B (Fungizone) are the most frequently employed antifungal agents. Both exert their fungicidal action by increasing the permeability of cell membranes in yeasts and fungi. Nystatin lacks any significant

TABLE 16.6 Commonly Employed Aminoglycoside Antibiotics with Comparative Ototoxicity and Nephrotoxicity Tendencies

Agent	Nephrotoxicity	Ototoxicity
gentamicin (Garamycin)	+ + +	+ +
tobramycin (Nebcin)	+ +	+ +
amikacin (Amikin)	+ + +	+ +
streptomycin	+	+ + +

untoward effects when administered topically and is the preferred agent for common fungal infections involving the skin, vagina, mouth, and remaining GI tract.

Amphotericin B causes many serious reactions, including reduced renal function in 80 percent of the patients treated! Although it may be employed topically, it is generally reserved for very serious infections and requires hospitalization for proper intravenous use.

SYNOPSIS OF THERAPEUTIC AGENTS

I. Sulfonamides

  A. ACTION
    1. Interrupt folic acid synthesis
  B. USES
    1. Urinary-tract infections
    2. Otitis media
  C. PREPARATIONS
    1. Gantrisin
    2. Septra
  D. SIDE EFFECTS
    1. Allergy
    2. Crystalluria

II. Penicillins

  A. ACTION
    1. Inhibit cell-wall synthesis
  B. USES
    1. Gram-positive cocci
    2. Syphilis and gonorrhea

II. Penicillins *(continued)*

    C. PREPARATIONS
        1. Narrow-spectrum
            a) penicillin G and V
        2. Broad-spectrum (to include some gram-negative organisms)
            a) ampicillin
        3. Penicillinase-resistant
            a) methicillin
    D. SIDE EFFECTS
        1. Allergy

III. Cephalosporins

    A. ACTION AND SIDE EFFECTS
        1. Same as penicillin
    B. USES
        1. Same as penicillin with extended gram-negative spectrum
    C. PREPARATIONS
        1. First generation—cephalexin (Keflex)
        2. Second generation—cefamandole (Mandol)
        3. Third generation—cefotaxime (Claforan)

IV. Erythromycins

    A. ACTION
        1. Inhibit ribosomal protein synthesis
    B. USES
        1. Penicillin-sensitive infections in patients allergic to penicillin
    C. BRAND PREPARATIONS
        1. E-mycin
        2. EES
    D. SIDE EFFECTS
        1. High incidence of nausea

V. Tetracyclines

    A. ACTION
        1. Inhibit ribosomal protein synthesis
    B. USES
        1. Broadest spectrum of activity

V. Tetracyclines *(continued)*

C. PREPARATIONS
 1. Tetracycline (Achromycin)
D. SIDE EFFECTS
 1. Phototoxicity
 2. Enamel staining

VI. Aminoglycosides

A. ACTION
 1. Inhibit ribosomal protein synthesis
B. USES
 1. Gram-negative bacilli
C. PREPARATIONS
 1. Gentamicin (Garamycin)
D. SIDE EFFECTS
 1. Ototoxicity—both vestibular and auditory
 2. Nephrotoxicity

VII. Antifungals

A. ACTION
 1. Alter cell-membrane permeability
B. USES
 1. Fungal and yeast infections
C. PREPARATIONS
 1. Nystatin (Mycostatin)

ARTICLES FOR DISCUSSION

1. **O'Donnell, J.** 1983. Antibiotic prophylaxis in surgical infection. *Heart and Lung* 12:20–22.
2. **Fernsebner, B.** 1982. Antimicrobial therapy for surgical patients. *AORN Journal* 36:479–486.
3. **Moss, J., et al.** 1982. A prospective drug utilization review on the prescribing of oral and parenteral cephalosporins. *Hospital Formulary* 17:1589–1600.
4. **Nicotra, M. B., et al.** 1982. Antibiotic therapy of acute exacerbations of chronic bronchitis: A controlled study using Tetracycline. *Annals of Internal Medicine* 97:18–21.

5. **Beam, J. R.** 1983. The new beta-lactam antibiotics. *Hospital Formulary* 18:44–52.

6. **Lamplet, J., and Habel, M. L.** 1981. The aminoglycoside antibiotics. *American Journal of Nursing* 81:1144.

7. **Eliopoulous, G. M., and Moellering, R. C.** 1982. Azlocillin, mezlocillin, and piperacillin: New broadspectrum penicillins. *Annals of Internal Medicine* 85:755–760.

8. **Genco, R. J.** 1981. Antibiotics in the treatment of human periodontal diseases. *Journal of Periodontology* 52:545–558.

9. **Rams, J. E., and Keyes, P. H.** 1983. A rationale for the management of periodontal diseases: Effects of Tetracycline on subgingival bacteria. *Journal of the American Dental Association* 107:37–41.

10. **O'Donnell, J.** 1983. Antibiotic prophylaxis in surgical infection. *Heart and Lung* 12:20–22.

REFERENCES

1. **American Heart Association.** 1977. Committee on Prevention of Rheumatic Fever and Bacterial Endocarditis. *Circulation* 56:139A–143A.

2. *Prophylaxis in Surgery,* Veterans Administration Ad Hoc Interdisciplinary Advisory Committee on Antimicrobial Drug Usage. 1977. *JAMA* 237:1003–1008.

3. **Crossley, K., et al.** 1981. Antimicrobial prophylaxis in surgical patients. *JAMA* 245:722–726.

4. **Goodman, L. S. and Gilman, A.** 1980. *The Pharmacological Basis of Therapeutics.* 6th ed. New York: Macmillan.

5. Ibid., p. 1156.

6. **Smith, C. R., et al.** 1980. Double-blind comparison of the nephrotoxicity and auditory toxicity of gentamicin and tobramycin. *New England Journal of Medicine* 302:1106–1109.

7. **Keys, T. F., et al.** 1981. Renal toxicity during therapy with gentamicin or tobramycin. *Mayo Clinic Proceedings* 56:556–559.

17

Antineoplastic Agents

Cancer is second only to cardiovascular disease as a cause of overall mortality in the United States. It is the leading cause of death for women aged 30 to 54 and children aged 3 to 14. Although surgical excision and radiation therapy are viable treatment modalities for localized or regionalized malignancy, they are hopelessly ineffective once the disease has disseminated. It is in this latter case that antineoplastic drugs can be of considerable use.

The antimicrobial agents, discussed in Chapter 16, have the advantage of interacting with structural and functional processes unique to microbial cells. Antineoplastic drugs are not as selectively toxic because tumor cells are actually derived from the host. Therefore, we are confronted with the sobering realization that "tumor-toxic" agents are very likely to exhibit toxicity toward normal cells as well. Adding to this rather dismal outlook is the fact that even a single cancer cell surviving chemotherapy may repopulate and eventually kill the host.

Most human cells undergo a growth cycle referred to as the "cell cycle." This cycle consists of five phases designated G_1, S, G_2, M, and G_0. Figure 17.1 illustrates this cycle and explains each of the phases. Most human tissues, including tumors, contain a variety of cells, all in various phases of this cycle. While individual cancer cells do not divide more rapidly than normal cells, most do spend a disproportionate amount of time in the M-phase of the cell cycle. For this reason, malignant tumors (cancer) grow more rapidly than other human tissue.

Most antineoplastic drugs act by disrupting cell cycles during the S and M phases. Predictably, human tissues containing cell populations which divide frequently are most susceptible to toxic effects from these drugs. The most common tissues affected are GI muscosa, bone marrow, and hair follicles. Table 17.1 lists the common effects experienced from toxicity to these particular tissues. Bone marrow suppression (myelosuppression) is the most common cause of morbidity and/or mortality and often severely limits drug dosage. For this reason, weekly blood counts are performed during the early course of treatment and eventually extended to three-week intervals.

Figure 17.1 The phases of the cell cycle.
Antineoplastic agents are most effective when acting at the S and M phases. The events occurring at each phase are:

G_0—Following mitosis (M), cells may stay inactive or dormant for periods of time.

G_1—RNA and protein synthesis takes place, providing cell growth.

S —Cell is committed to undergo division and begins to replicate its DNA.

G_2—DNA has been replicated, and the cell prepares to undergo mitosis.

M —The Cell undergoes the four stages of mitosis: prophase, metaphase, anaphase, and telophase.

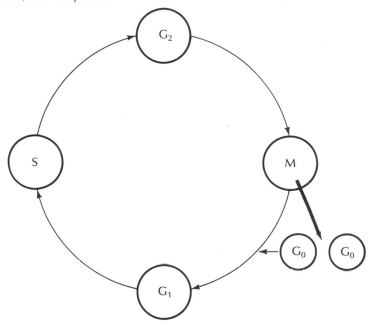

TABLE 17.1 Toxic effects of antineoplastic agents*

Gastrointestinal Toxicity	Bone Marrow	Epidermis
Nausea and vomiting	Anemia	Hair loss (alopecia)
Ulcerations	Leukopenia	Nail loss
Inflammation, for example, enteritis, gastritis, stomatitis	Granulocytopenia (agranulocytosis) Lymphopenia	Abnormal pigmentation
Hemorrhage	Thrombocytopenia	

*The most common toxic effects produced by the antineoplastic agents involve the GI tract, bone marrow, and epidermal structure.

ALKYLATING AGENTS

Agents belonging to this class exert their action by cross-linking DNA strands, rendering them nonfunctional in replication and protein synthesis. Since these effects bear a striking similarity to those produced by radiation therapy, alkylating agents are sometimes described as "radiomimetic agents." While they may exert this action at any phase of the cell cycle (cycle nonspecific), they are most effective during late G_1 and S phases. Of several agents found in this class, cyclophosphamide (Cytoxan) is the most commonly used. While all adverse effects listed in Table 17.1 are possible, hair loss (alopecia) is quite prominent. Noteworthy is the fact that this agent is not irritating to the skin of those handling the medication, or to the patient, should extravasation occur during IV administration.

ANTIMETABOLITES

Methotrexate is an analog of folic acid and thereby interferes with DNA synthesis. You may recall that the sulfonamides exert their antimicrobial action by interfering with the actual synthesis of folic acid. In contrast, humans obtain preformed folic acid in their diet which renders sulfonamides useless as antineoplastic agents. However, by competing as a false substrate, methotrexate is able to inhibit folic acid's role in DNA synthesis. Noteworthy is the high incidence of oral ulcerations and inflammation (stomatitis) associated with its use.

Since purines and pyrimidines are the nucleotides comprising DNA molecules, drugs which are analogs of these basic units are able to either block DNA synthesis or actually become an integral part of the DNA chain. In the latter case, the resulting DNA molecule is nonfunctional in coding the synthesis of vital proteins, such as enzymes. Fluorouracil (5-FU) and mercaptopurine are exemplary of this type of antimetabolite.

ANTIBIOTIC AGENTS

This antineoplastic class is named according to the strict definition of "antibiotic"—chemicals derived from microorganisms that are toxic against other cell types (in this case, tumor cells). These agents interfere with either DNA or RNA synthesis, depending on the particular agent. They are not selective enough in this action to be useful in antimicrobial therapy and therefore are employed solely as antineoplastic agents.

Doxorubicin (Adriamycin) is a commonly used member of this class. In addition to the toxicities common to most antineoplastic agents, doxorubicin produces a high incidence of cardiac toxicity leading to a severe form of congestive heart failure in which digitalis preparations are ineffective. This represents a grave situation in which the mortality rate exceeds 50 percent of those patients experiencing cardiac toxicity. Extravasation during intravenous administration produces considerable tissue inflammation and necrosis requiring immediate irrigation and other palliative measures.

Bleomycin (Blenoxane) is somewhat unique in that it produces little significant myelosuppression and is quite popular in combination regimens enabling lower dosage of those drugs which produce significant bone marrow suppression. Unfortunately its lack of marrow toxicity is somewhat offset by its high incidence of hypersensitivity and pulmonary fibrosis. This latter toxicity is most common in patients over age 70 and in those receiving heroic doses.

VINCA ALKALOIDS

Members of this class are derived from the plant, *Vinca rosea,* and act by inhibiting the formation of mitotic spindles. For this reason, the vinca alkaloids are considered cell-cycle specific (M-phase).

Vincristine (Oncovin) in combination with prednisone produces complete remission in up to 90 percent of children suffering acute lymphocytic leukemia. Vincristin produces little myelosuppression but frequently produces neurotoxicity, which initially manifests as parasthesia (partial numbness) and loss of tendon reflexes.

Like doxorubicin, the vinca alkaloids are very irritating to tissues, resulting in phlebitis and severe tissue sloughing should extravasation occur during intravenous administration.

STEROIDAL HORMONES

In Chapter 15 we discussed the many actions of the glucocorticosteroids. Among these actions is a depression of lymphocyte growth and function. For this reason, prednisone has proven useful, in conjunction with other agents, in treating certain leukemias and malignant lymphomas. In other types of cancer, these steroids may be used to counteract inflammatory side effects of other antineoplastic agents.

Sex steroids and their inhibitors offer one of the most selective modalities in the chemotherapy of neoplastic disease. Tumors involving reproductive organs are often hormone-dependent, hormone-responsive, or both.

Hormone-dependent tumors are those which require a specific hormone for growth. Breast cancer in premenopausal women is often dependent on estrogen, and prostate cancer in men may be equally dependent on androgens. Oophorectomy (ovary removal) and orchiectomy (testes removal) are generally regarded as effective forms of treatment in these cases. Tamoxifen (Nolvadex), which blocks estrogen receptors, is an alternative and is presently the treatment of choice in postmenopausal women with estrogen-dependent breast cancer.

Hormone-responsive tumors are those which regress when treated with specific hormones. Estrogens, progestins, androgens, and glucocorticosteroids have all been used with varying degrees of success. Since the effects of estrogens and androgens are often physiologically opposite, it is not surprising that tumors which are hormone-dependent on one steroid class may be hormone-responsive to the other. Prostate cancer is often responsive to estrogen and represents the preferred treatment for advanced cases.

COMBINATION THERAPY

The mechanisms, complications, and selection rationale for antineoplastic agents are quite complex, and agents are often selected empirically by oncologists, physicians who specialize in their use. It is important to appreciate that combinations of several agents may be necessary to achieve total or even partial remission in most cases.

Combination therapy is designed to employ agents with different mechanisms of action to assemble a synergistic regimen for tumor suppression. Doses of each agent in the regimen may be lower than if used alone and thus reduce the incidence of toxicity to the host. As an example, Table 17.2 lists the preferred regimen for Hodgkin's disease. Notice that each member of this regimen is from a unique class and varies from the others in the type and the frequency of toxic effects.

In summary, it is worth mention that the terms "effective" and "useful," when applied to antineoplastic drugs, are not so absolute as they are when applied

TABLE 17.2   MOPP regimen for treating Hodgkin's Disease

Agent	Class/Mechanism	Common Toxicity
mechlorethamine (Mustargen)	alkylating agent; cross-links DNA molecule	nausea and vomiting myleosuppression
vincristine (Oncovin)	Vinca alkaloid; inhibits mitotic spindle	neurotoxicity constipation
procarbazine	miscellaneous; not established	myelosuppression nausea and vomiting
prednisone	Glucocorticosteroid; depresses lymphoid tissue	cushingoid symptoms

to other drug classes discussed in this text. Whereas digitalis is described as "effective" in reestablishing myocardial contractility, antineoplastic drugs may be viewed as "effective" if they merely improve subjective symptoms or prolong life for a modest period.

Pharmacologists and other researchers have made impressive strides in developing antineoplastic agents. Unfortunately, their research is a most difficult challenge, and all will admit to its humbling nature.

ARTICLES FOR DISCUSSION

1. **Manni, A.** 1983. Hormone receptors and breast cancer. *New England Journal of Medicine* 309:1383.
2. **Bingham, C. A.** 1978. The cell cycle and cancer chemotherapy. *American Journal of Nursing* 78:1201.
3. **Chabner, B. A. et al.** 1975. The clinical pharmacology of antineoplastic agents. *New England Journal of Medicine* 292:1107–1113, 1159–1168.
4. **Jolivet, J., et al.** 1983. The pharmacology and clinical use of Methotrexate. *New England Journal of Medicine* 309:1094.
5. **Mar, D. D.** 1981. Antineoplastic drugs. *American Journal of Nursing* 81:1680–1683.
6. **Dreizen, S., et al.** 1975. Oral complications of cancer chemotherapy. *Postgraduate Medicine* 58:75–82.
7. **Bersan, G., and Carl, W.** 1983. Oral care for cancer patients. *American Journal of Nursing* 83:533–536.
8. **Cassileth, P., et al.** 1983. Antiemetic efficacy of Dexamethasone therapy in patients receiving cancer chemotherapy. *Archives of Internal Medicine* 143:1347–1349.
9. **Mattia, M. A., and Blake, S. L.** 1983. Hospital hazards: Cancer drugs. *American Journal of Nursing* 83:758–762.
10. **Reich, S. D.** 1981. Antineoplastic agents as potential carcinogens: Are nurses and pharmacists at risk? *Cancer Nursing* 4:500–502.

18

Agents Utilized in Respiratory Therapy

Many of the drug classes discussed throughout this text are used for the treatment of obstructive pulmonary diseases. The fundamental goal in this treatment is to improve the capacitance of the various duct systems comprising the respiratory tract. Simply stated, airway capacitance may be improved in three ways:

1. Relaxing the smooth muscle comprising duct walls.
2. Inhibiting inflammatory destruction and swelling of respiratory mucosa.
3. Eliminating mucosal secretions which "clog" the lumens.

SMOOTH MUSCLE RELAXANTS

The relaxation of bronchial smooth muscle is the most common goal attempted in the pharmacological management of respiratory disease. Beta-adrenergics and methylxanthines are the primary agents utilized, but anticholinergic agents are also gaining prominence. In Chapter 2 we discussed autonomic control of airway diameter (bronchioles) and saw that $beta_2$-receptor stimulation, as well as cholinergic-receptor (muscarinic) blockade, resulted in bronchial dilation.

> The activation of receptors on cell membranes of smooth muscle cells is merely the beginning of a complex series of chemical events which determine the intracellular availability of calcium ions. Following beta₂ receptor activation, a membrane-bound enzyme, adenylate cyclase, is activated and converts adenosine triphosphate (ATP) into cyclic 3',5'-*adenosine* monophosphate *(cyclic AMP)*. This so-called "second messenger" then activates a series of reactions leading to the efflux and the sequestration of calcium ions. The resulting lack of free calcium ions prevents smooth-muscle contraction (see Figure 18.1A).

Figure 18.1
Biochemical events leading to smooth-muscle contraction and relaxation. Bronchodilation may result by employing beta-receptor agonists, muscarinic-receptor antagonists, or phosphodiesterase inhibitors (PDI).

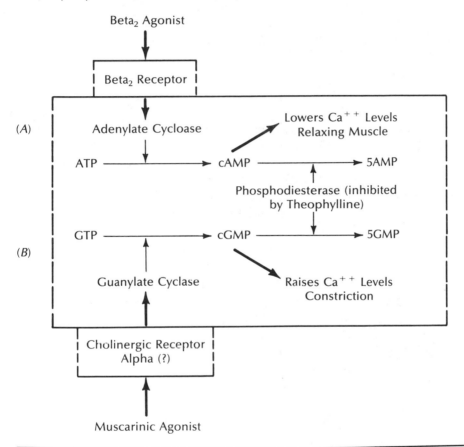

Following the activation of membrane-bound cholinergic receptors by either acetylcholine or muscarinic agonists, guanylate cyclase activity is increased, which leads to the formation of cyclic 3',5'-*guanosine monophosphate (cyclic GMP)*. This messenger then activates a series of reactions leading to elevated intracellular calcium levels and subsequent smooth muscle contraction. This same mechanism has been proposed following alpha-receptor stimulation but appears to be generally insignificant owing to the sparse alpha-receptor population on bronchial smooth muscle (see Figure 18.1B).

> Both cGMP and cAMP are metabolized by phosphodiesterase enzymes. Drugs which inhibit these enzymes—phosphodiesterase inhibitors (PDI) prolong the intracellular actions of these cyclic compounds. However, the methylxanthines appear to exhibit a greater inhibitory effect on enzymes inactivating cAMP than those enzymes which metabolize cGMP. In this manner, theophylline potentiates the relaxant action of cAMP more so than the constrictive action of cGMP.

BETA-ADRENERGICS

Beta-adrenergic agonists are the most commonly employed bronchodilator agents. Since cardiac stimulation due to beta$_1$ receptor stimulation poses the most serious side effects, efforts have been made to develop agonists with a more selective beta$_2$-receptor affinity. One must keep in mind that, despite the claims of some manufacturers, no agent can be heralded as ''perfect'' in beta$_2$-receptor affinity, and tachycardia must always be anticipated. Table 18.1 lists the beta agonists commonly used for bronchodilator therapy.

> Structural-activity relationships determining adrenergic-receptor affinity were addressed in Chapter 4. Structural relationships also play a role in determining the duration of action of these drugs by altering their susceptibility to enzymatic action. Resorcinols are not substrates for COMT and therefore, tend to be longer-acting than catecholamines. Substitutions on the nitrogen atom, as well as alpha carbon (next to the amine group), limit the compound's inactivation by MAO. It is for this latter reason that isoetharine is longer-acting than other catecholamines.

Tachycardia and CNS stimulation are the most common secondary (side) effects following beta-adrenergic therapy and are most often dose-related. However, three additional untoward responses are worth discussion.

Some patients experience a paradoxical bronchospasm following adrenergic therapy, especially with aerosol administration. Although no explanation has been accepted as conclusive, several have been proposed:

1. Metabolites of some compounds may function as beta-receptor antagonists and therefore block normal beta-mediated bronchodilation.
2. Dilation of lower airways may permit accumulation of secretions from upper airways.
3. Smooth-muscle relaxation may be so pronounced that compliance results in a ''collapse'' of the lumen.

TABLE 18.1   Comparisons of Beta Agonists Commonly Employed as Bronchodilators

Phenyl		Ethyl	Amine	Receptor Affinity Beta₂	Beta₁	alpha	Duration (hrs.) (Aerosol)

	Phenyl		Ethyl	Amine	$Beta_2$	$Beta_1$	alpha	Duration (hrs.) (Aerosol)
Catecholamines								
epinephrine	3, 4 = OH	OH		HCH₃	+ + +	+ + +	+ + +	.5-2
isoproterenol	3, 4 = OH	OH	H	CH(CH₃)₂	+ + + +	+ + + +	0	.5-2
isoetharine	3, 4 = OH	OH	C₂H₅	CH(CH₃)₂	+ + +	+	0	3-4
Resorcinols								
metaproterenol	3, 5 = OH	OH	H	CH(CH₃)₂	+ + +	+ +	0	3-4
terbutaline	3, 5 = OH	OH	H	C(CH₃)₃	+ + +	(+)0	0	3-7
Miscellaneous								
ephedrine	None	OH	CH₃	CH₃	+ + +	+ + +	+ +	3-4 (oral)
albuterol	3 = CH₂OH	OH	H	C(CH₃)₃	+ + + +	+	0	4-6

0 = no affinity   + to + + + + = progressively greater affinity

4. Aerosols are irritating and may trigger a reflex, vagal-induced constriction.

Though seldom clinically significant, a slight drop in PaO₂ may occur following bronchodilator therapy. This results from an upset in ventilation-perfusion ratios and may occur in one of two manners:

1. Relaxation of vascular smooth muscle offsets the normal physiological shunts observed around poorly ventilated alveolar units. Normally, vessels surrounding these units constrict in order to shunt blood towards better ventilated units.
2. Cardiac beta₁ stimulation may increase cardiac output, raising perfusion disproportionately to ventilation capabilities.

As stated above, this concept is seldom clinically relevant and can be offset by oxygen supplementation.

Tachyphylaxis is a term used to describe the rapid development of tolerance to any drug. In the case of bronchodilator therapy, the accumulation of beta-receptor–blocking metabolites or mucous plugs is a likely explanation. However, the tolerance following prolonged use of these agents must not be considered a tachyphylactic incident. There is ample evidence to support a reduction in the number of beta-receptors (down-regulation) following prolonged use of receptor agonists, and this offers the most tenable explanation.[1]

XANTHINE DERIVATIVES

At the present time, theophylline is the most common methylxanthine utilized clinically for the treatment of asthma, although caffeine has shown bronchodilator efficacy.[2] Theophylline inhibits the action of phosphodiesterase enzymes which inactivate cAMP. This has generally been regarded as the mechanism by which it relaxes bronchial smooth muscle.

> This mechanism is now questionable, considering the fact that phosphodiesterase is not significantly inhibited at the plasma concentrations achieved with normal therapeutic doses. The bronchodilation may be due in part to this action but may also be the result of prostaglandin inhibition or decreased release of histamine and leukotrienes from mast cells.
>
> Furthermore, the benefit a patient receives may not be entirely due to a bronchodilator effect. Theophylline has been found to increase diaphragmatic contractility and, in this manner, may improve the dyspnea and the respiratory weakness associated with bronchospastic disorders.[3]

Since beta-adrenergics stimulate cAMP formation and theophylline hinders its destruction, a natural synergism in bronchodilator action occurs with these two drug classes. Like beta-adrenergics, methylxanthines stimulate the myocardium and produce CNS stimulation which manifests as tremors, or convulsions if high doses are used. Their diuretic effect is due to the inhibition of sodium reabsorption and, in some cases, increased glomerular filtration resulting from increased cardiac output and vasodilation. Most of the side effects listed in Table 18.2 are more likely to occur when plasma levels exceed 20 mcg/ml. For this reason, intravenous therapy may require frequent monitoring of plasma theophylline levels.

> Therapeutic concentrations are from 10 to 20 mcg/ml and may be difficult to maintain because of wide variations in hepatic microsomal ac-

tivity. This variation in enzyme activity may be related to sex, age, health status, or concurrent therapy with other drugs that may induce or inhibit microsomal activity. Sustained-release formulations, such as Theo-Dur, represent a major advance in providing more consistent, prolonged plasma levels following oral administration.[3]

Since methylxanthines have a low solubility in water, agents used intravenously are actually salt preparations. Aminophylline is the most common agent used intravenously and is actually an ethylenediamine salt of theophylline (theophylline ethylenediamine). While it shares all the pharmacological properties of theophylline, it is only 79 to 86 percent equivalent in dosage. For example, a loading dose of 5.8 mg/kg of aminophylline is required to equal 5 mg/kg of anhydrous theophylline.[4]

TABLE 18.2   Theophylline's Side Effects*

CNS Stimulator	Cardiac Stimulation	Gastric Stimulation
restlessness	tachycardia	hyperacidity
nausea and vomiting	PVCs	
tremors		
convulsions		

*Stimulatory effects on the heart, stomach, and CNS account for theophylline's major side effects.

ANTICHOLINERGICS

Anticholinergic agents may provide striking improvement for those patients in whom cholinergic pathways are primarily responsible for increased smooth-muscle tone. Although dramatic claims have been reported for the atropine derivative, ipratropium (SCH 1000), it remains investigational in the United States. Despite numerous articles verifying anticholinergic efficacy, skeptics hesitate to employ them, citing fear of increased mucous vicosity and tachycardia as side effects. These fears may be more empirical than factual considering the positive results observed with glycopyrrolate (Robinul) which actually produces a greater degree of secretory inhibition than atropine.[5, 6] It appears likely that nebulized forms of either ipratropium or glycopyrrolate will eventually be used with greater frequency.

ANTI-INFLAMMATORY AGENTS

The inflammatory response, discussed in Chapter 15, plays a significant role in most pulmonary diseases. Not only do inflammatory mediators promote bronchospasm, but edema and swelling congest the entire respiratory tree. The release of mediators such as histamine and SRS-A from mast cells appears to the calcium dependent with cAMP functioning to inhibit their release. The entire system of membrane receptors, cyclase enzymes, and phosphodiesterase enzymes described for the contraction of smooth muscle also function to release mediators in the mast cell. Consistent with this arrangement, beta agonists, phosphodiesterase inhibitors (PDI), and anticholinergic agents not only relax smooth muscle, but inhibit mast-cell–mediator release as well.

Histamine Blockers and Cromolyn

Antihistamines and cromolyn are not actually classified as anti-inflammatory agents. However, considering the role of histamine and leukotrienes in the inflammatory respiratory diseases, their inclusion at this point seems appropriate.

The H_1 blockers (antihistamines), discussed in Chapter 15, have not proven useful in respiratory therapeutics. However, this is understandable when one considers that histamine is seldom the sole mediator responsible for bronchospasm or inflammatory congestion of passages.

Cromolyn sodium (Intal) has been found to be an effective prophylactic treatment for both allergic- and exercise-induced asthma. It prevents the release of histamine and SRS-A by a membrane stabilizing action on the mast cell, working independently of the cAMP system. It has few untoward effects other than coughing and irritation triggered by the powder form in which it is inhaled. It must be emphasized that this agent is not a histamine-receptor blocker and must never be considered an antihistamine. While antihistamines block histamine receptors, cromolyn prevents the *release* of mast cell products. Furthermore, from this action, it is obvious that cromolyn is only useful as a prophylactic agent. Once mast cell contents are released, evoking an acute condition, cromolyn is without beneficial action.

Steroidal Agents

Glucocorticosteroids are quite useful in the management of obstructive pulmonary disease. Not only do they potentiate the beneficial effects of catecholamines and PDIs in producing bronchodilation, but their anti-inflammatory actions reduce mucosal swelling and inflammatory destruction of respiratory tissues. Prednisone is the most commonly employed oral preparation and beclomethasone (Vanceril) is used only as an aerosolized preparation. Although all of the adverse effects discussed in Chapter 15 are possible, they are less likely following topical administration. However, aerosolized forms are more frequently associated with opportunistic infection, and this must be emphasized since oral and pharnygeal *Candida* infections following aerosolized forms of administration are fairly common.

The NSAIDS are of little use in the treatment of COPD. While some species of prostaglandins certainly contribute to the inflammatory process, the E-series (PGE) is quite protective to the respiratory tract. Not only do they relax bronchial smooth muscle, but they also function to inhibit mediator release from mast cells. In fact, the inhibitory action of aspirinlike preparations on prostaglandin synthesis may actually exacerbate COPD or precipitate bronchospasm in asthmatic patients. In contrast, the F-series of prostaglandins (PGF) are potent bronchoconstrictors; and inhibition of their synthesis may eventually prove useful. Unfortunately, at the present time, NSAIDS are not very specific in their inhibition of prostaglandin synthetase enzyme systems. However, the synthesis and the utilization of PGEs as actual bronchodilator agents is quite encouraging and may eventually be a welcome addition to our bronchodilator regimen.[7]

MUCOKINETIC AGENTS

The final topic to consider for improving obstructive disorders is the mobilization of airway secretions. Preparations utilized for this purpose may be collectively referred to as mucokinetic agents. The goals in this form of therapy are hydration and/or lysis of mucous plugs, thereby facilitating their removal.

Hydration Therapy

The hydration of airway secretions reduces their viscosity and thereby facilitates the expectoration of mucus. Since mucus normally contains 95 percent water, hydration is a logical modality to lesson its viscosity. Although distilled water may be used, it is more common to use isotonic or hypertonic saline solutions. When using these solutions one must not disregard the potential for sodium and water absorption which may prove hazardous for patients with congestive heart failure. Hypertonic solutions are irritating and may facilitate expectoration but the potential to induce bronchospasm may necessitate concurrent bronchodilator administration. In this regard, one should not dismiss the efficacy of PO and IV fluids in decreasing mucous viscosity and certainly eliminates the concern over topical irritation. It is worth emphasizing here that many drugs, taken for other disorders, are capable of increasing mucous viscosity as a side effect and, in themselves,

TABLE 18.3 Drugs Used for Conditions Other than Respiratory Disease which may Increase Mucous Viscosity*

Class	Example Preparations
Anticholinergics	atropine, benztropine (Cogentin)
Antihistamines	diphenhydramine (Benadryl)
Antipsychotics	haloperidol (Haldol)
	chlorpromazine (Thorazine)
Tricyclic antidepressants	imipramine (Tofranil)
	amitriptyline (Elavil)
	doxepin (Sinequan)
Certain narcotics	meperidine (Demerol)

*Due to anticholinergic activity.

may indicate the zealous use of hydration therapy. Some of the medications that may increase mucous viscosity as a side effect are listed in Table 18.3.

Mucolytic Agents

The major mucolytic agent employed in respiratory therapeutics is acetylcysteine (Mucomyst). It accomplishes its mucolytic action by cleaving the disulfide group in the mucoprotein molecule. This does not disrupt the protein portion but significantly lessens mucous viscosity by forming smaller subunits. This agent induces a significant incidence of bronchospasm, especially the more concentrated form (20 percent), and may require concurrent bronchodilator therapy. The ''rotten-egg'' odor of this agent is nauseating to many patients, and the therapist should be prepared to prevent aspiration should vomiting occur during its use.

Enzymatic destruction of purulent secretions may be accomplished with several enzyme preparations, but toxicity and questionable efficacy have limited their use. Deoxyribonuclease (Dornase) is a proteolytic enzyme which depolymerizes DNA chains. Since DNA found in necrotic cells comprising purulent exudate may increase the viscosity of the mucus, the use of Dornase would appear logical. However, it is not surprising that clinical reports have been unfavorable since the enzyme has no action on the mucoprotein component of mucus.

ARTICLES FOR DISCUSSION

1. **Gerrity, T. R., et al.** 1983. The effect of aspirin on lung mucociliary clearance. *New England Journal of Medicine* 308:139–141.
2. **Griffin, M., et al.** 1983. Effects of leukotriene D on the airways in asthma. *New England Journal of Medicine* 308:436–439.
3. **Weissmann, G.** 1983. The eicosanoids of asthma. *New England Journal of Medicine* 308:454–456.
4. **Weinberger, M., and Hendeles, L.** 1983. Slow-release theophylline: Rationale and basis for product selection. *New England Journal of Medicine* 308:760–764.
5. **Dusdieker, L., et al.** 1982. Comparison of orally administered metaproterenol and theophylline in the control of chronic asthma. *Journal of Pediatrics* 101:281–287.
6. **Spector, S. L.** 1983. The use of inhaled corticosteroid aerosols in the treatment of asthma. *Hospital Formulary* 18:421–426.
7. **Wolfe, J. D., et al.** 1978. Bronchodilator effects of terbutaline and Aminophylline alone and in combination in asthmatic patients. *New England Journal of Medicine* 298:363–367.
8. **Sahn, S. A.** 1978. Corticosteroids in chronic bronchitis and pulmonary emphysema. *Chest* 73:389–396.
9. **Webb, J., et al.** 1982. A comparison of the effects of different methods of administration of beta$_2$ sympathomimetics in patients with asthma. *British Journal of Diseases of the Chest* 76:351–357.
10. **Shapiro, G. G., et al.** 1983. Double-blind evaluation of methylprednisolone versus placebo for acute asthma episodes. *Pediatrics* 71:510–514.
11. **Isles, A. F., and Newth, C. J. L.** 1983. Combined beta agents and methylxanthines in asthma. *New England Journal of Medicine* 309:432.
12. **Wilson, J. D., and Sutherland, D.C.** 1982. Combined beta agents and methylxanthines in asthma. *New England Journal of Medicine* 307:1707.
13. **Adinoff, A. D., and Hollister, R.** 1983. Steroid-induced fractures and bone loss in patients with asthma. *New England Journal of Medicine* 309:265.
14. **Mathewson, H. S.** Intravenous Aminophylline: A dangerous therapeutic weapon. *Respiratory Care* 27:713–715.
15. **Pak, C. F., et al.** 1982. Inhaled atropine sulfate: Dose-response characteristics in adult patients with chronic airflow obstruction. *American Review of Respiratory Diseases* 125:331–334.
16. **Mathewson, H. S.** 1983. Bronchoactive autacoids and their antagonists. *Respiratory Care* 28:1175–1177.

17. **Mathewson, H. S.** 1983. Risks and benefits of aerosolized steroids. *Respiratory Care* 28:325–326.
18. **Mathewson, H. S.** 1983. Anticholinergic aerosols. *Respiratory Care* 28:467–468.
19. **Bruderman, I., et al.** 1983. A comparative study of various combinations of ipratropium bromide and metaproterenol in allergic asthma patients. *Chest* 83:208.
20. **Braigelman, W.** 1984. Here come the anticholinergics (editorial). *Chest* 85:297.

REFERENCES

1. **Motulsky, H. J., and Insel, P. A.** 1982. Adrenergic Receptors In Man: Direct identification, physiologic regulation, and clinical alterations. *New England Journal of Medicine* 307:18–29.

2. **Becker, A. B., et al.** 1984. The bronchodilator effects and pharmacokinetics of caffeine in asthma. *New England Journal of Medicine* 310:743–746.

3. **Isles, A. F., et al.** 1982. Theophylline: New thoughts about an old drug. *Chest* 825:49s–54s (Supplement).

4. **AMA Division of Drugs.** 1943. *AMA Drug Evaluations*, 5th ed. Philadelphia: W.B. Saunders, p. 591.

5. **Gal, T. J., and Surett, P. M.** 1981. Atropine and glycopyrrolate effects on lung mechanics in normal man. *Anesthesia and Analgesia* 60:85–90.

6. **Johnson, B. E., et al.** 1984. Effect of inhaled glycopyrrolate and atropine in asthma. *Chest* 85:325–328.

7. **Weissman, G.** 1983. The eicosanoids of asthma. *New England Journal of Medicine* 308:454–456.

19

Pharmacological Aspects of Cardiac Emergencies

Many of the allied health professions perform vital roles in the care of patients suffering a variety of acute cardiac disorders. The American Heart Association has made admirable strides in training health professionals in basic and advanced cardiac life support.[1] Certification in these programs is becoming a standard for improving the quality of emergency care inside and outside our health care facilities.

A substantial portion of emergency cardiac care depends on the rational use of pharmacotherapeutic agents. Most of these agents have been introduced in preceding chapters, and it is hoped that the reader will consider all of those topics prerequisite to the contents of this chapter.

HYPOXEMIA AND ACIDOSIS

The sine qua non of emergency care is oxygen delivery to the tissues. For the patient in cardiac arrest, this must be accomplished by adequate ventilation and cardiac compressions (CPR). If we fail in our attempt to ventilate and perfuse the tissues, remaining therapeutic options will prove ineffective in an environment of combined respiratory and metabolic acidosis. In this setting, sodium bicarbonate is valuable for converting metabolic acids, such as lactic acid, to carbonic acid. However, elevated carbonic acid levels will leave the patient in a state of respiratory acidosis unless adequate ventilation is performed to eliminate carbon dioxide (Figure 19.1). However, one must not be overzealous in the use of sodium bicarbonate since this may produce complications equal in gravity to acidosis. Sodium and water overload, alkalosis, and impaired oxygen release from hemoglobin are some of the complications which can be avoided by proper ventilation and bicarbonate utilization. Until test results on blood gases are available, sodium bicarbonate should be administered as a 1mEq/kg loading dose, followed every 15 minutes by half this initial dose.

Figure 19.1
Sodium bicarbonate converts metabolic acids (lactic-H) to carbonic acid by exchanging a sodium atom for a hydrogen atom. The carbonic acid must then be eliminated by expiring carbon dioxide. Therefore, adequate ventilation is critical for total conversion of metabolic, as well as respiratory acidosis.

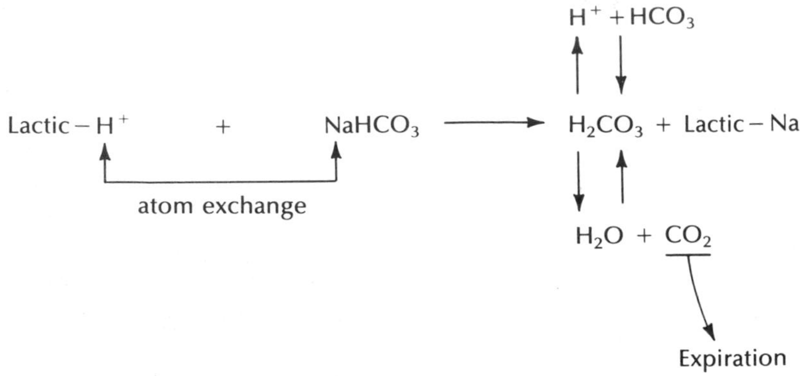

$$H^+ + HCO_3$$

$$Lactic - H^+ \quad + \quad NaHCO_3 \longrightarrow H_2CO_3 + Lactic - Na$$

atom exchange

$$H_2O + CO_2$$

Expiration

ADRENERGIC AGONISTS

As discussed in Chapter 4, the effects produced by adrenergic agonists depend primarily on their affinity for specific adrenergic-receptor types. The primary goals of these agents in cardiac emergencies is to increase tissue perfusion by improving cardiac function and arterial pressure. Beta agonists are able to increase heart rate, atrioventricular conduction, and myocardial contractility. These actions improve cardiac output and elevate systolic blood pressure. In contrast, alpha agonists are used to elevate diastolic pressure by their vasoconstrictive action. One should remember that all adrenergic agonists increase myocardial oxygen consumption, again stressing the vital importance of ventilation during resuscitative efforts. The inotropic and chronotropic effects produced by beta agonists are primary determinants of oxygen consumption while alpha-receptor–induced vasoconstriction increases the effort for cardiac ejection (afterload).

Epinephrine is the adrenergic agent most utilized in cardiac arrest, regardless of the underlying electrocardiographic rhythm. Its beta-receptor action stimulates contractility in asystole or electromechanical dissociation (EMD) and facilitates defibrillation efforts in ventricular fibrillation. The alpha-adrenergic effect on vascular tone is also considered beneficial for the ultimate restoration of cardiac function and explains the preference for epinephrine over isoproterenol as an initial drug selection.[2] Epinephrine is generally administered in .5 to 1 mg doses by the intravenous route although sublingual injection or endotracheal tube instillation are valuable alternatives should a vein not be accessible (Table 19.1).

TABLE 19.1   Typical concentrations, doses, and routes of administration of epinephrine (Note that 1:1000 concentrations must never be injected intravenously.)

Preparation	Total Amount	Route & Dose
1 ml vials	1 mg	.5 ml (.5 mg) subcutaneous*, sublingual
10 ml syringe 1:10,000	1 mg	5 ml (.5 mg) IV, sublingual
		10 ml (1 mg) intratracheal**

---

*This route is not very effective with the poor perfusion typical in cardiac arrest. However, it is the preferred route for treating major allergic reactions and asthmatic attacks.
**Following injection into the lumen of the endotracheal tube, positive pressure is initiated to force the solution down the respiratory tract.

Isoproterenol is the most potent nonspecific beta-receptor agonist and is indicated in asystole, EMD, and third-degree heart block. In all of these conditions, the administration of isoproterenol should follow unsuccessful attempts with either epinephrine and/or atropine. By blocking the inhibitory action of the parasympathetic system on the heart, atropine may permit the sympathetic correction of asystole and AV block. Should this prove ineffective, adrenergic stimulation with isoproterenol is indicated (see Table 19.2).

Dopamine is established as a useful agent in many hypotensive conditions, as well as in cardiogenic shock. In addition to its ability to stimulate alpha and beta receptors, its affinity for dopaminergic receptors provides excellent renal perfusion. The dose-response characteristics of dopamine were presented in Chapter 4 and should be mastered before using this agent. It is indicated for hypotensive episodes following conversion from initial cardiac dysfunctions. Typically this follows conversion from cardiac arrest, bradycardia, and/or AV block.

Dobutamine is a catecholamine derivative possessing selective beta$_1$-receptor affinity. It is unique in that it has a major effect on contractility (inotropy) with only a minimal effect on heart rate (chronotropy). Its inotropic effect is comparable to that of digitalis although the mechanism of action differs. Its major advantages over glycoside preparations are its rapid onset, brief half-life, and relative lack of cardiac toxicity compared to glycosides. Dobutamine is particularly useful for improving cardiac output and systolic pressure in heart failure following myocardial infarction.[3]

Other vasopressor agents—alpha-adrenergics, may be used if the above agents are unsuccessful in stabilizing hemodynamic status. However, these agents

TABLE 19.2 Recommended sequence in the *pharmacological* management of specific cardiac emergencies (in cardiac arrest, ventilation and sodium bicarbonate therapy must be initiated along with these agents[1])

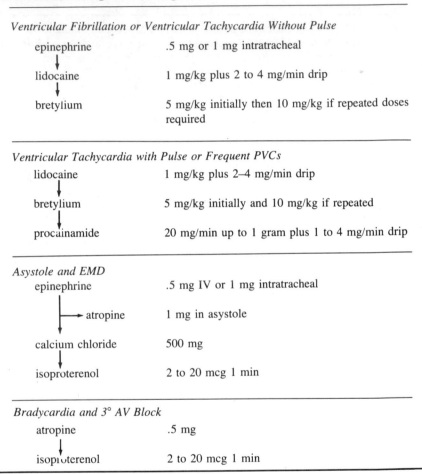

Ventricular Fibrillation or Ventricular Tachycardia Without Pulse

epinephrine	.5 mg or 1 mg intratracheal
lidocaine	1 mg/kg plus 2 to 4 mg/min drip
bretylium	5 mg/kg initially then 10 mg/kg if repeated doses required

Ventricular Tachycardia with Pulse or Frequent PVCs

lidocaine	1 mg/kg plus 2–4 mg/min drip
bretylium	5 mg/kg initially and 10 mg/kg if repeated
procainamide	20 mg/min up to 1 gram plus 1 to 4 mg/min drip

Asystole and EMD

epinephrine	.5 mg IV or 1 mg intratracheal
atropine	1 mg in asystole
calcium chloride	500 mg
isoproterenol	2 to 20 mcg 1 min

Bradycardia and 3° AV Block

atropine	.5 mg
isoproterenol	2 to 20 mcg 1 min

are seldom primary selections and offer few advantages over the actions of epinephrine, isoproterenol, and dopamine in acute care situations.

ANTIDYSRHYTHMIC AGENTS

As explained in Chapter 7, action potentials (impulses) in cardiac conductive tissues are initially generated by the influx of either sodium or calcium ions (see Figure 19.2). The primary agents utilized to treat cardiac dysrhythmias act by

Figure 19.2
Action potentials of ventricular *(A)* and atrial *(B)* neuroconductive cells. Note the major roles of sodium (Na) and calcium (Ca) ions in generating the action potentials.

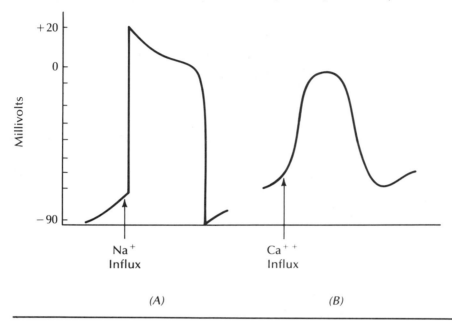

blocking the inward flow of these ions and therefore serve to stabilize the conductive membranes which generate dysrhythmic activity.

Lidocaine is the drug of choice for treating virtually all ventricular dysrhythmias. These include ventricular fibrillation and tachycardia, as well as a variety of premature ventricular contractions (PVCs).

> Caution must be exercised to rule out sinus bradycardia and AV block as primary causes of PVC genesis. In this case, atropine's positive influence on heart rate may provide a correction of the ectopic pacemaker activity. In the setting of total heart block, lidocaine's depressant action on ventricular tissue may eliminate the ability of this tissue to assume its role as an escaped pacemaker.

Lidocaine has a brief plasma half-life owing to rapid hepatic biotransformation. For this reason, bolus injections must be followed by continuous infusion to sustain therapeutic blood levels. The most common dosage schedule utilized in treating any of the ventricular dysrhythmias mentioned above is 1 mg/kg loading dose, followed by an infusion rate ranging from 1 to 4 mg/min.

> The most common sequel to myocardial infarction is ventricular fibrillation. Since lidocaine has been shown to elevate the fibrillation threshold of ventricular tissue, there is considerable interest in the prophylactic use of lidocaine for patients suffering an infarction. On this basis, many emergency-room physicians recommend lidocaine to prevent cardiac arrest in the myocardial infarction setting. While the American Heart Association has not taken an official stand on the issue, they do recommend lidocaine following conversion from ventricular fibrillation to help prevent its recurrence.

A "tingly or numbing" sensation, referred to as parasthesia, is the most common side effect produced by intravenous lidocaine. Convulsive seizures may be precipitated when high blood levels of lidocaine develop following repeated boluses or poor hepatic perfusion in the pump-failure setting. Drowsiness and disorientation will usually warn of this impending emergency and may indicate lidocaine withdrawal. Diazepam is usually effective in terminating seizure activity should it occur.

Procainamide is quite similar to lidocaine in action and is indicated in those dysrhythmias unresponsive to lidocaine. Since it is more likely to produce hypotension and excessive depression of conductive tissues than lidocaine, hypotension and widening of the QRS complex are indications for discontinuing its use. Like lidocaine, it is short-acting and requires a continuous drip (1 to 4 mg/min) after the dysrhythmia is suppressed with slow intravenous doses (20 mg/min) up to 1 gram.

Bretylium has gained prominence in the treatment of ventricular dysrhythmias that are refractory to lidocaine. Its actions are quite complex and must be separated into antidysrhythmic and hemodynamic categories. It raises the fibrillation threshold and depresses dysrhythmic activity by a variety of poorly understood mechanisms. Significant, however, is the fact that it prolongs the refractory period of normal ventricular tissue, making it less susceptible to stimulation by neighboring excitable foci (reentrant pathways). In addition to this antidysrhythmic action, bretylium produces two paradoxical effects on sympathetic nerves. Initially it stimulates catecholamine release which may result in dysrhythmogenic and hypertensive effects sometimes referred to as "sympathetic storm." Within 15 to 20 minutes it blocks the further release of catecholamines, resulting in a hypotensive effect. While these hemodynamic actions are not so significant when using bretylium to facilitate defibrillation of a patient in cardiac arrest, they are cause for concern when using it to correct PVCs and ventricular tachycardia in a patient with a functional hemodynamic status. In this latter setting, some physicians prefer to maintain a concurrent lidocaine drip to protect the heart during the initial dysrhythmogenic period of bretylium administration.

Propranolol, while fairly effective, has limited use in the treatment of ventricular tachycardia and PVCs. As a beta antagonist, it is able to block sympathetic stimulation of ectopic foci; but this same action may be quite perilous in the potential setting of myocardial failure. Without hemodynamic monitoring, for example, Swan-Ganz catheterization, to establish left ventricular function, propranolol may lessen myocardial contractility. Its major use occurs in dysrhythmias refractory to the above agents, especially digitalis toxicity. In this case, the beneficial inotropic effect of digitalis is not exerted through beta-receptor mechanisms and is not reversed by propranolol.

At the present time, verapamil is the major calcium channel blocker employed for the treatment of paroxysmal atrial tachycardia (PAT). Unpredictable responses occur when it is used for atrial flutter and fibrillation, thus retaining digoxin as the preferred agent for these latter conditions. Since calcium channel blockade may decrease myocardial contractility, pump failure is a possible adverse effect in compromised settings. Diltiazem appears to produce less negative inotropic action and may eventually replace verapamil in PAT therapy.

In addition to its role in neuroconductive tissue, calcium influx is crucial for smooth-muscle contraction. This renders calcium channel blockers quite useful for vasodilator therapy. Their ability to dilate coronary arteries, and their peripheral vasodilating properties which reduce preload and afterload, make these agents useful in the ischemic and heart failure settings. Table 19.3 compares the hemodynamic and cardiac actions of the calcium channel blockers, nitrates, and beta blockers. Specific uses of nitrate preparations will be discussed later in this chapter.

TABLE 19.3   Cardiovascular effects of selected cardiac drugs*

Agent	Vasodilation	Nodal Depression	Negative Inotropy
nifedipine (Procardia)	+ + +	+	+ ,0
verapamil (Isoptin)	+	+ +	+ +
diltiazem (Cardizem)	+	+	+ ,0
nitroglycerin	+ + +	0	0
beta blockers	0	+ +	+ +

+ = mild
+ + = significant
+ + + =
*This table compares the cardiovascular effects of three calcium channel blockers, nitrates, and beta blockers.[4, 5]

Verapamil is administered in doses of .1 mg/kg up to 10.0 mg over a 2 to 3 minute period. The patient's hemodynamic status should be closely observed, which is true for all drugs administered intravenously.

Since results of calcium blockade have been addressed, it seems appropriate to discuss the role of "calcium addition" in emergency cardiac care. Following the depolarization of cardiac muscle, intracellular calcium levels increase and provide the fundamental link in driving the contractile apparatus. For this reason, the administration of calcium ions, in the form of calcium chloride, is indicated to improve myocardial contractility in the presence of asystole or EMD. Since calcium also plays an active role in the action potential of conductive tissues, it may worsen other dysrhythmias and is intended only to improve contractility in the absence of cardiac ejection. It is actually contraindicated in ventricular fibrillation since it may create a situation refractory to defibrillation.

NARCOTIC THERAPY

The analgesic, sedative, and hemodynamic effects of narcotic agents renders them very useful for patients suffering myocardial infarction or congestive heart failure. Their benefit in treating the pain and the anxiety of these conditions is obvious, but the hemodynamic benefits must not be underestimated. By several mechanisms, including depression of the vasomotor control center, arterial and venous dilation results in a blood-pooling effect in the abdominal tissues. This results in a decreased venous return (preload) and, to a lesser extent, a decrease in afterload. This action is of obvious benefit to an ischemic myocardium and is equally advantageous in reducing the pulmonary congestion associated with left-side heart failure. While morphine is most commonly employed, meperidine and nalbuphine are comparable in efficacy. The latter agent has gained popularity due to its decreased tendency for producing respiratory depression. Although hypotension and respiratory depression are hazards of narcotic therapy, slow administration, while observing for signs of slurred speech and drooping eyelids (ptosis), serve as safe end points. Doses of morphine and nalbuphine may range anywhere from 2 to 20 mg, thus stressing the need for careful titration.

NITRATE THERAPY

As discussed in Chapter 8, the mechanism by which nitrate preparations relax smooth muscle is poorly understood. However, they are particularly effective on vascular smooth muscle and vary somewhat in their predilection towards venous rather than arterial dilation.

There is no doubt that nitroglycerin can dilate coronary arteries, but in patients suffering arteriosclerotic forms of coronary disease, this effect is unlikely. It is generally accepted that peripheral venous dilation accounts for nitroglycerin's ability to relieve the pain of angina pectoris, thus reducing preload and, hence, myocardial oxygen consumption. While arteriolar dilation may occur, afterload reduction is not so nearly pronounced as venous dilation. Arteriolar dilation is more evident following intravenous infusion than with sublingual tablets, which is equally true regarding the dilation of coronary arteries.

Sublingual nitroglycerin tablets will generally relieve the pain of angina pectoris in 3 to 5 minutes. This is so consistent that, should pain persist following three doses, myocardial infarction is the likely diagnosis. Hypotension is not frequent in a supine position, but if it should occur, reflex tachycardia is of major concern in an ischemic setting.

Sodium nitroprusside produces dilation in both veins and arteries, thereby reducing myocardial preload and afterload. Its action is most useful in hypertensive crisis and acute congestive failure. In this latter situation, nitroprusside combined with dopamine, dobutamine, or digoxin has proven quite effective in stabilizing hemodynamic status.

DIURETIC THERAPY

Pulmonary edema is a major consequence of left-heart failure. This condition, as well as any other incidence of excessive fluid retention, is an indication for the use of diuretic therapy. Furosemide (Lasix) is the agent of choice and is administered in intravenous doses of .5 to 2 mg/kg. The onset of diuresis is rapid (5 minutes) and reaches its peak in approximately 30 minutes. This rapid volume depletion may complicate hemodynamic status, necessitating close observation of blood pressure.

SUMMARY

Emergency cardiac care concentrates on the stabilization of ischemic episodes, cardiac dysrhythmias, blood pressure, and congestive heart failure. Since pump failure is prevalent by itself, or following myocardial infarction, many of these agents have been described in terms of positive effects in this situation. Three primary goals in the pump failure setting are diuresis, improved myocardial contractility, and reduction in myocardial workload (preload and afterload). Table 19.4 summarizes those agents which reduce preload and afterload forces on the failing myocardium. Table 19.2 summarizes the indications and the dosages of agents recommended by the American Heart Association in the delivery of advanced cardiac life support.

TABLE 19.4 Comparative effects on preload and afterload of agents commonly employed for cardiac emergencies

Agents	Preload	Afterload
diuretics	+ +	0 (+)
narcotics	+ +	+
Nitroglycerin (sublingual)	+ +	0 (+)
Nitroglycerin (IV)	+ +	+
nitroprusside	+ +	+ +

+ = mild
+ + = significant

ARTICLES FOR DISCUSSION

1. **Mathewson, H. S.** 1982. Drugs for prevention of sudden death. *Respiratory Care* 27:1536–1539.
2. **Rossi, L. P., and Antman, E. M.** 1983. Calcium channel blockers: New treatment for cardiovascular disease. *American Journal of Nursing* 83:382–387.
3. **Purcell, J. A.** 1982. Shock drugs: Standardized guidelines. *American Journal of Nursing* 82:965–974.
4. **Roberts, J. R., et al.** 1979. Blood levels following intravenous and endotracheal epinephrine administration. *Journal of the American College of Emergency Physicians* 8:53–56.
5. **Wyman, M. G., and Gore, S.** 1983. Lidocaine prophylaxis in myocardial infarction: A concept whose time has come. *Heart and Lung* 12:358–361.
6. **Lee, G., et al.** 1981. Hemodynamic effects of morphine and nalbuphine in acute myocardial infarction. *Clinical Pharmacology and Therapeutics* 29:576–581.
7. **Gal, T. J., et al.** 1982. Analgesic and respiratory depressant activity of nalbuphine: A comparison with morphine. *Anesthesiology* 57:367–374.
8. **Brown, D. C., et al.** 1979. Asystole and its treatment: The possible role of the parasympathetic nervous system in cardiac arrest. *Journal of the American College of Emergency Physicians* 8:448–452.
9. **Braunwald, E.** 1977. Vasodilator therapy—A physiological approach to the treatment of heart failure. *New England Journal of Medicine* 297:331–332.
10. **Thal, E. R., et al.** 1979. Self-administered analgesia with nitrous oxide. *JAMA* 242:2418–2419.

REFERENCES

1. **American Heart Association.** 1983. *Textbook of Advanced Cardiac Life Support.*

2. **Yakaitis, R. W., et al.** 1979. Relative importance of alpha- and beta-adrenergic receptors during resuscitation. *Critical Care Medicine* 7:293–296.

3. **Goldstein, R. A., et al.** 1980. Comparison of digoxin and dobutamine in patients with acute infarction and cardiac failure. *New England Journal of Medicine* 303:846–849.

4. **Braunwald, E.** 1982. Mechanism of action of calcium channel blocking agents. *New England Journal of Medicine* 302:1618–1627.

5. **Antman, E. M., et al.** 1980. Calcium channel blocking agents in the treatment of cardiovascular disorders. *Annals of Internal Medicine* 93:875–885, 886–904.

20

Fluorides and Dental Medicaments

In addition to many of the systemically administered drugs already discussed, dental health care delivery utilizes many agents placed topically on oral tissues. Most outstanding is the use of topical fluorides for the purpose of reducing the occurrence of dental caries.

Fluoride is a very reactive element that is seldom found in its neutral atomic form. Rather, it is found throughout our environment, generally as fluorspar (CaF_2) or other mineral salts. In water, fluoride salts ionize into free fluoride ions (F^-) and are most prevalent in underground waters where contact with fluoride containing minerals is more likely. Therefore, our food, water, and even the air we breathe contains at least trace amounts of fluoride. Indeed the plasma fluoride levels are approximately .1 to .2 ppm (ppm = parts per million = grams per million milliliters) in areas where water supplies are not fluoridated.

Fluoride is mainly absorbed through the gastrointestinal wall, although trace amounts may be absorbed through the lungs and the skin. Following absorption, fluoride is distributed throughout most body tissues but is primarily stored in mineralized tissues as calcium fluoride or fluorapatite. Approximately 50 percent of an ingested dose will be excreted in the urine. Figure 20.1 illustrates the general pharmacokinetic pattern of the fluoride ion. There is little question that fluoride is the most impressive prophylactic agent in the prevention of dental caries. However, the exact mechanism by which fluoride exerts this anticaries effect is not firmly established. At the present time there are three schools of thought regarding this issue. They are discussed in the following three paragraphs.

Fluoride is able to replace hydroxyl ions in hydroxyapatite crystals at the enamel surface following systemic as well as topical administration (see Figure 20.2). The fluoroapatite crystal is less soluble in acids produced by bacteria as the initial step in cariogenesis. However, other substances have been identified which reduce the acid solubility of enamel but do not reduce the incidence of caries.

206

Figure 20.1 Pharmacokinetic pattern of fluoride: absorption, distribution, and excretion.

ABSORPTION
GI TRACT
LUNGS SKIN
PLASMA
BONE TEETH
SOFT TISSUES
GINGIVAL FLUID
URINE
FECES SWEAT

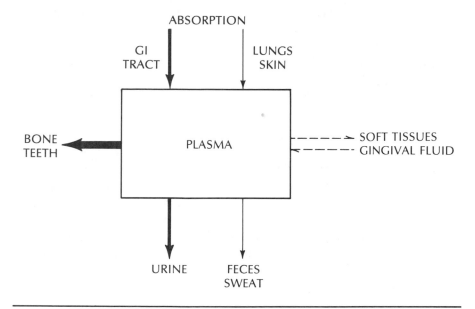

Figure 20.2

A. Fluoride ion replaces hydroxyl ions in hydroxyapatite. Fluoroapatite is more resistant to the erosive action of acids produced by cariogenic bacteria.

B. In high concentrations, fluoride may form calcium fluoride. This compound may then ionize, providing a continued source of fluoride to form additional fluoroapatite crystals.

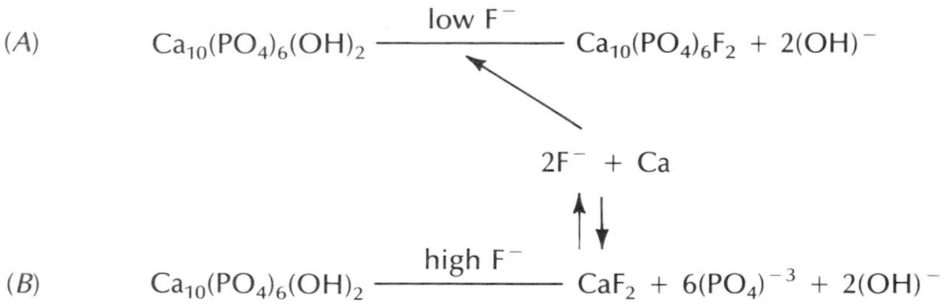

(A)
$Ca_{10}(PO_4)_6(OH)_2$
low F^-
$Ca_{10}(PO_4)_6F_2 + 2(OH)^-$
$2F^- + Ca$
(B)
$Ca_{10}(PO_4)_6(OH)_2$
high F^-
$CaF_2 + 6(PO_4)^{-3} + 2(OH)^-$

Fluoride ion inhibits bacterial enzyme systems. This not only results in a modest bacteriocidal effect but appears to reduce bacterial acid production. A smaller drop in pH occurs when fluoridated plaque is incubated in sucrose medium than when nonfluoridated plaque samples are used.

Fluoride ions promote the remineralization of surface enamel with calcium and phosphate ions during acid challenge. This concept, along with the fact that gingival fluid fluoride concentrations approximate those of plasma, is receiving considerable emphasis by researchers and may eventually prove to be the primary manner in which fluoride accomplishes its anticaries effect.

In high amounts, fluoride ion is quite toxic and is used in several rodenticides and insecticides. Unfortunately, this fact has helped nurture naive attitudes regarding its safe use in community water supplies. The acute lethal dose of fluoride is approximately 7 to 14 mg/lb. To place this in perspective, fluoridated water supplies are designed to contain 1 ppm fluoride ion. If you were to drink one liter of water a day, you will have consumed only 1 mg of fluoride! Following the ingestion of large amounts of fluoride tablets or rinses, acute toxicity may occur, resulting from the ion's ability to inhibit several enzyme systems vital in cellular respiration reactions. Toxicity initially manifests as excessive salivation, abdominal pain, diarrhea, nausea, and vomiting. As fluoride ion exerts its calcium-binding effect, various neurological and skeletal muscle dysfunctions occur and ultimately culminate in convulsive seizures, respiratory depression, and/or cardiovascular collapse. Should an accidental overdose be suspected, milk or other calcium-containing product should be administered to bind any fluoride not yet absorbed. If toxic symptoms begin to present, intravenous calcium salts, such as calcium chloride or calcium gluconate, should be administered and preparation made to support respiration and cardiovascular function until an emergency squad can transport the patient to the nearest emergency room.

Chronic fluoride toxicity is subtle in onset and eventually manifests as enamel mottling in developing teeth or osteosclerosis, which may become debilitating in its most severe form. While mild enamel mottling may occur in developing teeth following daily consumption of water containing 1.6 ppm of fluoride, erupted teeth are not affected with this disorder. There is radiographic evidence of osteosclerosis with daily consumption of water containing 8 ppm, but crippling forms of this disorder require the daily ingestions of 20 to 80 mg of fluoride over a period of 10 to 20 years.[1]

Fluoridated water supplies appear to be the most effective fluoride delivery system for the population as a whole. However, in regions where the water supply is not fluoridated, the American Dental Association's Council on Dental Therapeutics has recommended a daily dosage schedule for systemic fluoride supplementation (see Table 20.1). Systemic fluoride administration is presently considered more important during years of tooth development although newer theories regarding gingival fluid fluoride levels may begin to alter this concept.

The topical application of fluoride is useful in reducing caries incidence as well as root sensitivity. Many systems are available including rinses, gels, and toothpastes. Approximately 90 percent of toothpastes marketed in the United

TABLE 20.1   Recommendations for daily dose of systemic fluoride administration to children*

Age	Fluoride Levels in Local Water Supply		
	< .3 ppm	.3 - .7 ppm	> .7 ppp
0-2	.25 mg	0	0
2-3	.50 mg	.25 mg	0
3-14	1 mg	.5 mg	0

*These recommendations are based on the amount of fluoride in the water supply (2.2 mg NaF = 1 mg F).

States contain fluorides. In most of these, there is 1 mg of fluoride per gram of toothpaste, which is the typical amount placed on a toothbrush at each brushing. Although typically viewed as a topical form of administration, one should not rule out therapeutic and toxic effects that may result from swallowing. It has been estimated that children may swallow 20 to 40 percent of the toothpaste used in each brushing!

Stannous fluoride (SnF) application is an effective caries-prevention formula which also exerts a caries-arrestment effect. Following application, large amounts of calcium fluoride are formed, which eventually provide fluoride for fluoroapatite formation. The phosphate ions freed during this calcium fluoride formation combines with the stannous ion to form insoluble tin-phosphate complexes. These complexes may impart an objectionable light-brown pigmentation to decalcified carious or precarious lesions. However, the insoluble nature of this complex provides a caries-arrestment effect and indicates the use of SnF in patients with high caries activity. The short shelf-life and meticulous administration technique required for the formulation makes its routine use unpopular for all patients.

Research has shown that fluoride uptake by enamel is increased when the pH of the solution is low. This concept provided for the introduction of acidulated phosphate fluoride (APF) preparations. While they do not impart any caries-arrestment action, they are superior to SnF in other aspects, such as higher enamel uptake, long shelf-life, and more agreeable taste. APF gel is the most popular fluoride formula used for professional application and may also be applied daily by patients experiencing a high caries index, since daily APF application has shown a significant reduction in the number of S. mutans in occlusal plaque samples.[2] Since fluoride does exert a bacteriocidal action, interest has developed regarding its daily use to inhibit those microorganisms implicated in periodontal disease. At the present time, research is inconclusive, but SnF appears to be more effective than APF preparations.

When applying the various topical regimens, the professional should be aware of the amount of fluoride contained in the preparation. This is of obvious value should a child inadvertently swallow a topical rinse or gel. Table 20.2 should prove useful in making this calculation for the particular brand preparation utilized.

TABLE 20.2 Fluoride content of commonly employed topical fluoride compounds.*

Compound		Amount Containing 1 mg F	mg F in 1 ounce
NaF	.05%	4.3 ml	6.5
	.20%	1.0 ml	25.5
	.22%	1.0 gm	28.3
	2.72%	.08 ml	348.1
MFP	.76%	1.0 gm	28.3
SnFl$_2$	.40%	1 gm	28.3

*Adapted from Whitford, G. M., Dental Hygiene 57:16–29 (1983).

DENTAL MEDICAMENTS

On the shelves and in the cabinets of the typical dental office is a multitude of tiny bottles containing various medicaments for topical use. While some of these may be used topically on the mucous membranes, such as steroids and local anesthetics, the majority are used in the treatment of dental tissues.

The most typical aroma in a dental office is attributed to eugenol, which is the principal ingredient in oil of cloves. It is a phenol derivative and, as such, possesses antiseptic properties by virtue of precipitating cellular protein. Its anodyne action (topical analgesia) often masks its irritating properties, which consistently initiate an inflammatory response in the soft oral tissues. Its most frequent use is as a solvent for zinc oxide powder in the formulation of cements, pastes, and dressings referred to as zinc oxide–eugenol (ZOE). This compound is useful for a variety of purposes listed in Table 20.3.

Many additional derivatives of phenol are used for their antiseptic action in treating pulpal and periapical tissues during endodontic treatment (root-canal therapy). Formocreosol is the most widely used of these agents and contains orthocresol and formalin (40 percent formaldehyde). The formaldehyde component is claimed to "mummify" pulpal tissues, preventing their breakdown products from

TABLE 20.3 Uses for zinc oxide–eugenol preparations in dental therapeutics

Temporary restorations	Treatment of localized osteitis (dry
Temporary cementation of crowns	socket)
Bases for large restorations	Bite registrations
Impressions	Periodontal dressings

acting as chronic inflammatory irritants. Table 20.4 illustrates the various phenol derivatives used as intracanal medicaments in endodontic therapy.

Calcium hydroxide is a compound historically used to stimulate pulpal tissue (odontoblasts), to form reparative dentin in deeply carious teeth. It has also

TABLE 20.4 Derivatives of phenol utilized as dental medicaments

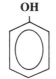

PHENOL

Single-Entity Agents

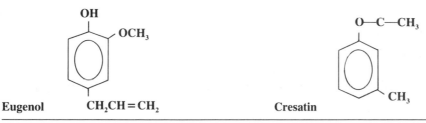

Eugenol $CH_2CH=CH_2$ **Cresatin**

Mixtures

Parachlorophenol   and   Camphor   = Camphorated Parachlorophenol (CPC)
Crystals

Orthocresol   **and**   **Formaldehyde**   = **Formocrcosol**
(**Formalin**)

gained extensive use in endodontic therapy for the purpose of stimulating the closure of open-root apices. The mechanism by which this simple compound stimulates such a dramatic effect on dentin formation is unknown.

It would be tempting to assume that the calcium from the compound provides a mineral source for dentin and cementum formation. However, this is not the case, and studies examining high pH as a mechanism have proven equally fruitless. Nevertheless, its efficacy and low toxicity make calcium hydroxide a very useful agent. Indeed, this compound, along with the various phenol derivatives, comprise the most commonly employed topical medicaments in dental therapeutics.

ARTICLES FOR DISCUSSION

1. **Wei, S. H. Y.** 1975. Effect of topical fluoride solutions on the enamel surface as studied by scanning electron microscopy. *Caries Research* 9:445–458.
2. Editorial. 1981. Will the manufacturer of the best fluoride dentifrice please stand? *Journal of the American Dental Association* 102:958.
3. **Ripa, L. W.** 1981. Fluoride rinsing: What dentists should know. *Journal of the American Dental Association* 102:477–481.
4. **Ogard, B., et al.** 1980. Plaque-inhibiting effect in orthodontic patients of a dentifrice containing stannous fluoride. *American Journal of Orthodontics* 78:266–272.
5. **Tinanoff, N., et al.** 1980. Effect of stannous fluoride mouthrinse on dental plaque formation. *Journal of Clinical Periodontology* 7:232–241.
6. **Whitford, G. M.,** 1983. Fluorides: Metabolism, mechanisms of action, and safety. *Dental Hygiene* 57:16–29.
7. **Horwitz, H. S.** 1977. Misuse of topically applied fluoride. *Journal of Preventive Dentistry* 7:15–16.
8. **Shern, R. J., et al.** 1977. Enamel biopsy results of children receiving fluoride tablets. *Journal of the American Dental Association* 95:310–314.
9. **Gangarosa, L. P.** 1981. Iontophoretic application of fluoride by tray technique for desensitization of multiple teeth. *Journal of the American Dental Association* 102:50–52.
10. **Hastreiter, R. J.** 1983. Fluoridation conflict: A history and conceptual synthesis. *Journal of the American Dental Association* 106:486–493.

REFERENCES

1. **Holroyd, S. V., and Wynn, R. L.** 1983. *Clinical Pharmacology in Dental Practice*. 3rd ed. St. Louis: C. V. Mosby, p. 288.

2. **Loesche, W. J., et al.** 1975. Effect of topical acidulated phosphate fluoride on percentage of *Streptococcus mutans* and *Streptococcus sanguis* in plaque. *Caries Research* 9:139–155.

Index

Note: **(t)** means drug is listed in a table on the page noted.